IMAGES
of America

THE SEEING EYE

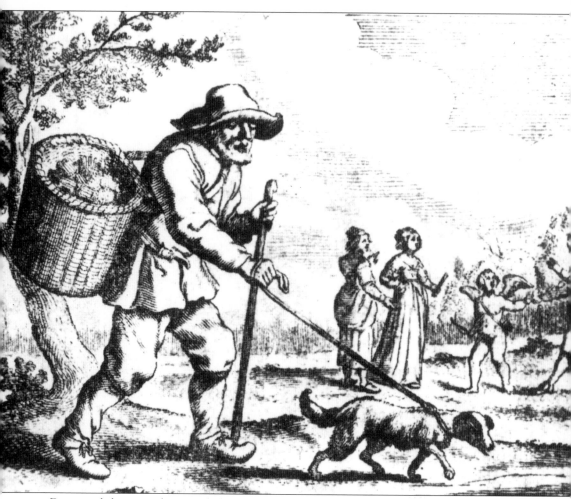

Dogs and humans have cohabited for more than 10,000 years. Sometime into the relationship—no one is exactly sure when—canine companions started serving as guides for people who were blind and visually impaired. There are some clues, however, as to when the partnership began. A painting on a wall of a house in Pompeii that was buried in the devastating volcano of A.D. 79 suggests that dog guides existed during the times of the Roman Empire. A scroll painting c. 1250 shows a man being guided by a dog through a crowded street in China. This European drawing dates from 1639. It illustrates a man with his dog on the end of a rigid leash. *Textbook for Teaching the Blind*, written in Austria by Fr. Johann Wilhelm Klein in 1819, notes that a rigid connection allows the person to feel when a dog is making a side movement or standing still, something that a soft leash cannot accomplish. Poodles and shepherds were the father's dogs of choice. In the United States, there are several written accounts from the mid-1800s that talk about dogs helping to guide their blind masters.

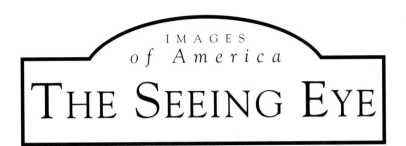

IMAGES
of America

THE SEEING EYE

Steve Swanbeck

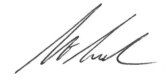

ARCADIA

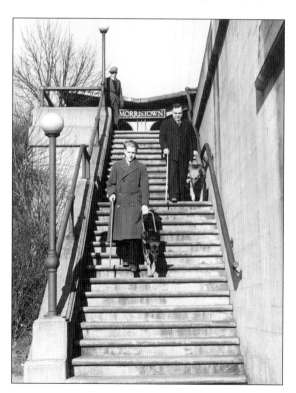

Morristown has served as an effective training ground for The Seeing Eye for nearly three quarters of a century. A train station staircase could be a challenge for anyone who is blind or visually impaired, but these two men and their German shepherds descend the steps with confidence. (Courtesy The Seeing Eye and Brown Brothers.)

CONTENTS

ACKNOWLEDGMENTS

This book was made possible as a result of the efforts of countless good people who have devoted themselves to the challenge of improving the lives of those who are blind and visually impaired. In the beginning, there were the pioneers with a vision. Supporting them were the exceptional dogs with the rare characteristics that are necessary to serve as the eyes for people who cannot see.

Over the years, the list of those who should be recognized continues to grow. There are Seeing Eye employees who, in all likelihood, could command greater salaries in other endeavors but choose this work because they have more profound motivations. There are volunteers who give freely of their time in many different capacities. There are benefactors who provide the financial backing necessary to make sure the program continues and that no one who qualifies for a dog guide is turned away for lack of resources.

Of course, the blind and visually impaired Seeing Eye graduates and students have taken on the biggest challenge. Only a small percentage of those who could benefit from a dog guide choose to do so. Their efforts and their example make it possible for others to follow.

There is not enough room here to acknowledge each individual, so thanks very much to all of you for sharing this glimpse of The Seeing Eye.

All of the photographs and documents in this book were culled from the extensive archive at The Seeing Eye and are the property of The Seeing Eye. Photographers who were identified with specific photographs are credited in parentheses at the end of the corresponding caption. Many thanks to all of the photographers whose work appears in this book.

Several additional sources of reading for those who are interested in The Seeing Eye include: *First Lady of The Seeing Eye*, by Morris Frank and Blake Clark; *Love in the Lead*, by Peter Brock Putnam; and *Dogs Against Darkness*, by Dickson Hartwell. They were helpful references for this book.

INTRODUCTION

There are places in this world where extraordinary things are accomplished. The Seeing Eye is one such place.

Settled comfortably atop one of the rolling hills of historic Washington Valley in Morris Township, New Jersey, The Seeing Eye is headquartered in a fitting location. During the winters of 1777 and 1779–80, during our nation's struggle for independence, Gen. George Washington made his headquarters a few miles from where organization is today. In the 21st century, Washington Valley remains the site of ongoing struggles. This is where some 300 people who are blind or visually impaired come each year and strive to regain a measure of their own independence.

The history of The Seeing Eye began in Europe in the 1920s. A well-to-do Philadelphia woman and her family moved to Switzerland to set up a breeding and training facility for German shepherd dogs. Dorothy Harrison Eustis raised dogs not for show but instead as working dogs that were intelligent, strong, and responsible. She entered into a partnership with a noted American trainer and geneticist named Jack Humphrey. Together they developed their own scientific approach to breeding and training.

During her ongoing research, Eustis learned of several schools in Germany that taught dogs to guide German veterans who were blinded in World War I and others who were visually impaired. She visited a school in Potsdam and was so impressed that she wrote an article about the school for the *Saturday Evening Post*. Published on November 5, 1927, the article was entitled "The Seeing Eye." The idea of a blind person being led across busy streets by a dog was greeted with skepticism by most people. Still, a 20-year-old blind man from Nashville, Tennessee, jumped at the chance to regain some of the independence he had lost three and a half years earlier. His name was Morris Frank, and he had the desire and confidence that would soon spark the inception of The Seeing Eye.

Although Eustis had no plans to get into dog guiding, she changed her mind after receiving a letter from Frank stating his interest. Eustis, husband George, and Humphrey researched the Potsdam program, made some modifications, and then trained several German shepherds to guide humans. When the dogs were ready in April 1928, they sent for Frank.

In Mount Pelerin, Switzerland, at the Eustis compound called Fortunate Fields, Frank met the first-ever Seeing Eye dog. She was a beautiful German shepherd that he named Buddy. Frank, Buddy, Humphrey, and George Eustis undertook a six-week training program that resulted in the bonding of a blind man and his dog. As a team, they navigated busy streets, dangerous stairways, crowded shops, and nearly anything else that lay ahead. Frank's struggle for independence had been won.

It was decided in Switzerland that a dog guide school would be established in North America. The Seeing Eye was incorporated in Nashville on January 29, 1929, and the first class began there in February. This was a bold undertaking. Most people were dubious, especially those connected with organizations for the blind. American culture was not keen on the idea of dogs joining people in restaurants, retail stores, trains, hotels, planes, and so on. There was no funding, and the nation's economy was about to nose-dive. Trainers were needed, and it took an exceptional person to become a trainer. Dogs were needed; they, too, had to be special. The Seeing Eye also required qualified students, those who could measure up to the task and prove to the skeptics that dogs could, in fact, serve as guides for blind people. These were a few of the major obstacles.

It was no small endeavor, indeed, for a small group of visionaries who believed they could offer people who were blind the opportunity to achieve greater independence, dignity, and self-confidence through the use of a Seeing Eye dog. Slowly, however, things came together. Several classes graduated with success. The Seeing Eye started to gain acceptance among its doubters. Summers in Nashville turned out to be too hot for this type of work, so the school relocated to Whippany, New Jersey, in 1931. The Seeing Eye administrator who was also a primary breeder, Willi Ebeling, lived in nearby Dover, New Jersey, and recommended the area. There were no extremes in the weather, and the town of Morristown, a few miles away, provided an ideal training environment.

The Seeing Eye grew and prospered in Whippany for more than 30 years. Eventually, the facility became outdated, so The Seeing Eye sold it and relocated to its present Morris Township campus in 1965. The work there continues. Since 1929, some 13,000 dog guides have been matched with blind and visually impaired men and women from the United States and Canada. The Seeing Eye is a philanthropy that receives no government aid of any kind. Private donations have funded the operation since it began.

The Seeing Eye is an important part of American history—an example of freedom, independence, vision, and courage.

One

A Young Man's
First Kiss

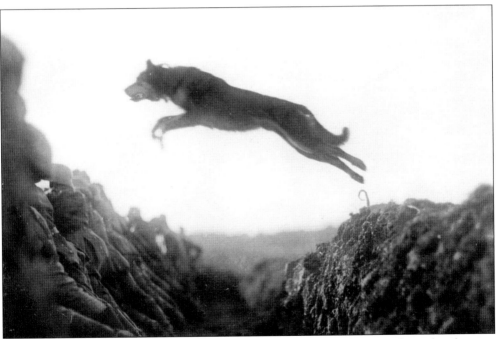

Dogs were employed to carry vital messages during World War I. They were faster than humans and just as reliable. After the war, Germany trained dogs to guide its blinded veterans. An inquisitive American woman learned of the German training program and developed a dog guide plan of her own that resulted in the founding of The Seeing Eye.

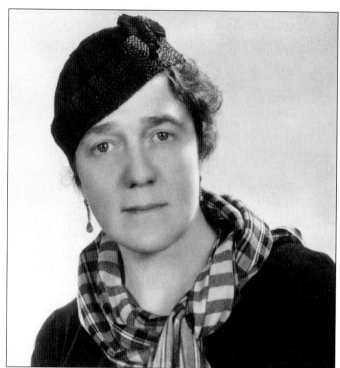

Dorothy Harrison was the youngest of six children born to a prominent Philadelphia family in 1886. She married at the age of 20 and had two sons. Several years later, she became interested in cattle breeding and then the breeding of German shepherds. She was widowed at 29 and, eight years later, married George Eustis. In 1923, the Eustis family moved to a small village called Mount Pelerin, which overlooked Vevey, Switzerland. There they established a breeding and training kennel for German shepherds called Fortunate Fields.

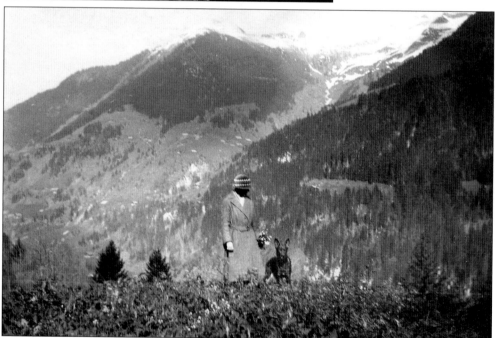

In this majestic setting, Dorothy (shown here in 1924) and George Eustis bred and trained German shepherds to become good working dogs. (It is noteworthy that Dorothy was sincerely dedicated to the project. George was a good trainer but more of a free spirit.) Although dogs have served in a working capacity for thousands of years, much breeding in the last century has focused on appearance versus performance.

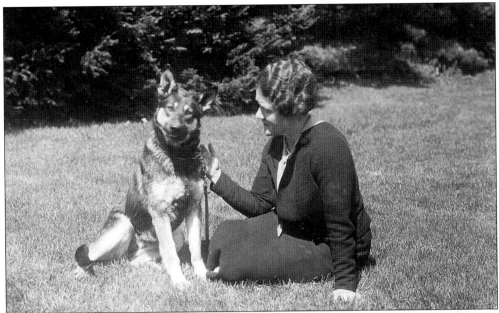

After they had been weaned, Fortunate Fields puppies were sent to live with farming families so that they would grow up with the benefit of human contact. At around 14 months, the puppies were brought back to Fortunate Fields for training. A similar policy is still in place today at The Seeing Eye. Dorothy Eustis is shown here with an eager young shepherd. (Courtesy The Seeing Eye and the Parker Studio.)

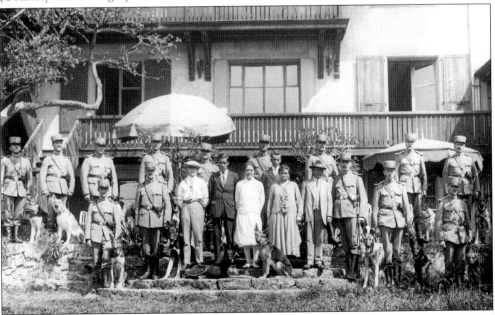

Dogs that were bred for their superior mental and physical abilities attracted the attention of the Swiss army and police. Soon, Fortunate Fields was training dogs, soldiers, and policemen. Dogs were used for patrolling, rescue, message carrying, sentry duty, and trailing. Dorothy and George Eustis are shown in the center of this photograph with students at Fortunate Fields in the 1920s. (Courtesy The Seeing Eye and A. Dauer.)

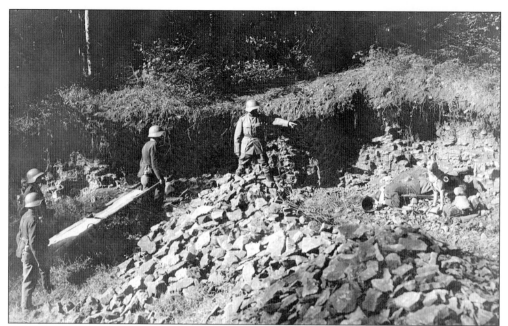

Some Red Cross dogs were trained to scout battlefields and find wounded soldiers. Once located, the dog would return to its Red Cross station and lead a rescue party back to the victim. A Red Cross logo can be seen on the Fortunate Fields shepherd shown here during a training exercise.

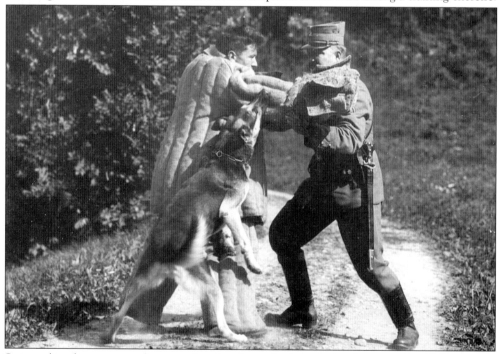

Swiss police dogs were used to apprehend and guard criminals (as shown in this 1928 training exercise at Fortunate Fields), to quell altercations, and to find missing persons. The shepherds were not vicious; they were taught to release their grip immediately upon the master's command or as soon as the criminal stopped resisting. (Courtesy The Seeing Eye and A. Dauer.)

Elliott S. "Jack" Humphrey was invited to Fortunate Fields by Dorothy Harrison Eustis in 1924 and was made a working partner. She learned of him after reading articles he wrote for the *Shepherd Dog Review* on the genetics and breeding of German shepherds. Born in Saratoga Springs, New York, Humphrey was an accomplished animal trainer and breeder. Among many other things, he worked with U.S. cavalry horses during World War I.

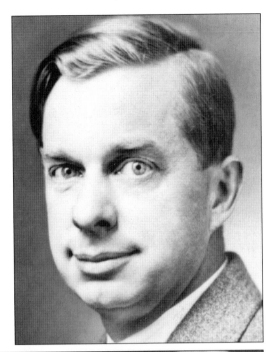

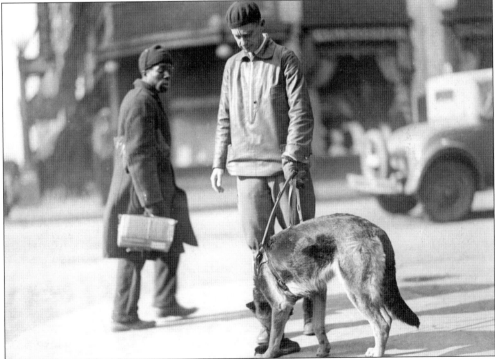

Humphrey (shown here teaching Gala to pick up a dropped article) and the Eustises created and developed a method of breeding dogs for intelligence, temperament, strength, and stamina. They wanted to produce dogs that would be of service to society. Humphrey brought a scientific approach to breeding and training, carefully studying the mental and physical characteristics required for good working dogs.

THE SEEING EYE

By
Dorothy Harrison Eustis

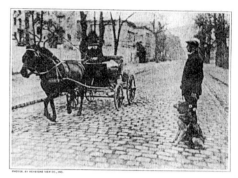

TO EVERYONE, I think, there is always something particularly pathetic about a blind man. Shorn of his strength and his independence, he is a prey to all the sensitiveness of his position and he is at the mercy of all with whom he comes in contact. The sensitiveness, above all, is an almost insuperable obstacle to cope with in his fight for a new life, for life goes on willy-nilly and the new conditions must be reckoned with. In darkness and uncertainty he must start again, wholly dependent on outside help for every move. His other senses may rally to his aid, but they cannot replace his eyesight. To man's never failing friend has been accorded this special privilege. Gentlemen, I give you the German shepherd dog.

Because of their extraordinary intelligence and fidelity, Germany has chosen her own breed of shepherd dog to

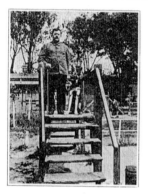

help her in the rehabilitation of her war blind, and in the lovely city of Potsdam she has established a very simple and businesslike school for training her dogs as blind leaders. Inclosed in a high board fence, the school consists of dormitories for the blind, kennels for the dogs and quarters for the teachers, the different buildings framing a large park laid out in sidewalks and roads with curbs, steps, bridges and obstacles of all kinds, such as scaffoldings, barriers, telegraph poles and ditches—everything in fact that the blind man has to cope with in everyday life.

Many Dogs and No Fights

THREE forces work together to make this school the model that it has become: The German Government, the Shepherd Dog Club of Germany and the association of war-blinded soldiers. The latter is a splendid organization of some 3000 men which strives continually and successfully to keep its members in work and above pity or charity and out of the class of beggars and peddlers. The government furnishes the land for the school and further grants each blind man a subsidy for his dog's keep after he has left the school.

The dogs are supplied by the Shepherd Dog Club of Germany and are either donated or bought at the lowest price compatible with the qualities they must have, for these blind leaders are the distant cousins and the cinderellas of famous show dogs; they not only have the goods but they deliver them in the shape of courage, intelligence and service. The total cost of a dog, trained and ready to leave the school, is about sixty dollars, which includes the initial cost of the dog.

They must be young and healthy, with quiet, steady nerves and a good character. As a whole, they are a very nice looking lot, especially when you take into consideration that not more than ten or twelve dollars has been paid for one of them. Moreover, they have a certain expression in their eyes, a sturdiness and interest which is too often lacking in their fashionable cousins. As the qualities of courage and intelligence are characteristics of the German shepherd dog wherever he is found unspoiled by intensive show breeding, it is not so hard to collect groups of these leaders for the blind as it would seem, and after a few simple tests to prove he is fit for the service, the new recruit can go to work, and all his work is founded on obedience.

> Now these are the Laws of the Jungle,
> And many and mighty are they;
> But the Head and the Hoof of the Law,
> And the Haunch and the Hump, is—Obey!

It is little short of marvelous how a raw dog can be taken into the school and in four months be turned out a blind leader, and the miracle is that the dog so perfectly

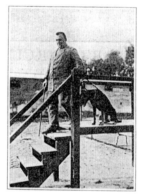

assimilates his instruction. From the very small beginnings of becoming absolutely house-broken, he is taken step by step upward to his life work of leading a blind man, of being that man's eyes and his sword and buckler. He is first let loose to run with all the other dogs and to learn to mind his P's and Q's and not to fight.

For any dog full of life and energy, this first step is an education in itself and of itself starts him thinking. After he has mastered his lesson, the park becomes a schoolroom; and here, with dogs running loose, people passing in all directions, laughing and talking, he has his first studies in concentration and learns to sit and lie down on command, to speak, to fetch, to carry; and he must learn good will and to do it all cheerfully, gladly and with dispatch. This is the A B C, or kindergarten, of obedience, and if he is an

apt pupil he learns it easily and graduates into the next class. Here he begins his work in the leading harness, which is more easily seen in the pictures than explained in words. He now learns that although he can romp with other dogs and exercise he can romp with other dogs in the park, from the moment the harness is put on him dogs must be anathema to him. Called from his play, a dog advanced in his work is ridiculously like a business man called to his office; you can almost see him lay aside his newspaper, settle his coat, straighten his necktie and take on an air of business affairs.

Life in a Big City

IN THE beginning, all schooling went on in the park; but it was soon found that a dog might work perfectly there and be of no use in the bustle and distraction of a city, so the park was given over to obedience exercises and the advanced classes were moved into the city itself. From the moment a dog wears the leading harness his schooling is done under actual working conditions. He must go at a fast walk so that the slackening in his gait for an obstacle is instantly felt through the rigid handle of his harness. For curbs he pulls back and stands still so that his master can find the edge with his cane; for steps, approaching traffic and all obstacles barring progress, he sits down; and for trees, letter boxes, scaffoldings, pedestrians, he

(Continued on Page 45)

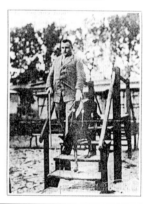

This article—written by Dorothy Harrison Eustis and published in the *Saturday Evening Post* on November 5, 1927—together with the response letter from Morris Frank on the next page set off a chain of events that led to the establishment of The Seeing Eye. Eustis reported on a school she visited in Potsdam, Germany, that trained dogs to guide war veterans and others who were blind. Filled with emotion when she saw what was achieved by the students and their canine companions, she wrote of the new independence that was experienced: "And then comes the whole great realization that the future holds freedom. No longer a care and a responsibility to his family and friends, he can take up his life where he left it off; no longer dependent on a member of the family, he can come and go as he pleases; and as these thoughts and possibilities gather strength in his mind, despair and loneliness give way to happiness and companionship."

THE NATIONAL LIFE AND ACCIDENT INSURANCE CO., Inc.

Nashville, Tenn.
November 9, 1927

Miss Dorothy Harrison Eustis
c/o Curtis Pub. Co.
Independent Sq.
Philadelphia

My dear Miss Eustis:

In reference to your article "The All Seeing Eye" which appeared in the Saturday Evening Post of Nov. 5th, is of great interest to me so that is the reason why I take the liberty to address this letter to you.

I have often thought of this solution for the blind but have never heard of it being put to a practical use before, of course there are a few cases throughout the United States realizing that if handled in the proper manner and supervised correctly this would be quite a help to the blind of our country. I would appreciate very much if you would be kind enough to give me more information upon this matter and if you would give me the address of this school in Germany, or of any trainer in this country who might have any thing similar as I should like very much to forward this work in this country, as three and a half years ago at the age of sixteen I was deprived of my sight and know from practical experience what rehabilitation means and what it means to be dependent upon a paid helper who are unsympathetic and not interested in their work and do not appreciate kindness as shown to them and as you well know that there are many throughout the land who not even have paid attendants.

I should like very much to be able to express my personal thanks and appreciation for the way in which you handle and put your message across. It touched those in my condition more knowing that what you said was near the real truth and I do believe that this gave the seeing public a very good idea of the situation and I hope it will help the public to come to a more clearer understanding as we do not require sympathy but a laughing word and a pat upon the back, kindly excuse me for rambling on in this manner but in my feeble way I am trying to give you the thanks you deserve.

Thanking you in advance for any information you may be able to let me have.

I remain sincerely yours,

Morris S. Frank
National Life and Accident Ins. Co.
National Bldg.
Nashville, Tenn.

When Morris Frank's father read him the *Saturday Evening Post* article in their living room in Nashville, the 20-year-old who was blind knew that his life had changed forever. "I tossed and turned all night," he explained years later. "One of these extraordinary animals could be the answer to my prayers. He could ease the bitterness I felt at losing my sight. I visualized myself walking freely down the street. I would be able to make calls on prospective clients for my insurance business without the encumbrance of a talkative, incompatible guide. I could go to college on my own. I could even have a date—and it would not have to be a double date." Frank was determined to get a dog guide, so he wrote this letter to Eustis on November 9, 1927, to find out how to do so.

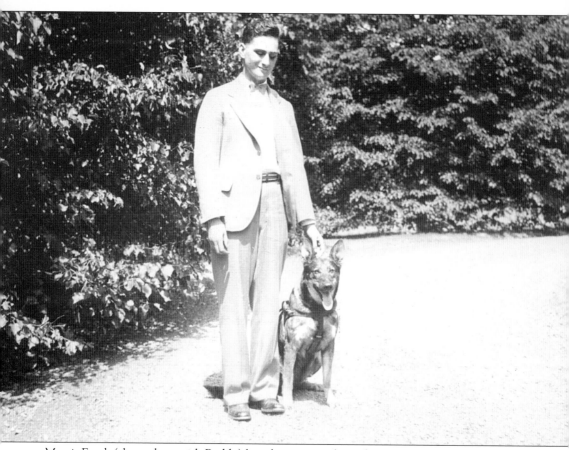

Morris Frank (shown here with Buddy) lost the vision in his right eye at age six when he ran into a tree limb while riding a horse. When he was 16, his left eye was blinded during a boxing match. Sadly, his mother had also been blinded in both eyes during two separate incidents. The audacious young man yearned for his independence, and Fortunate Fields might offer the solution. Following months of correspondence, Eustis agreed to train a dog guide for Frank, a new undertaking at Fortunate Fields. In April 1928, Frank sailed alone to Switzerland. Due to the norms at the time that considered blind people helpless, he was classified as a parcel by the shipper. The restrictions he endured during the voyage angered the young Tennessean, who eventually made it to the Continent more determined than ever to overcome his dependency on others. At Fortunate Fields, Frank met the first-ever Seeing Eye dog. She was a beautiful German shepherd named Kiss. Since it was impossible to envision himself strolling through downtown Nashville saying, "Here, Kiss. Come, Kiss," Frank promptly renamed his new companion Buddy.

Frank and Buddy can be seen taking some of the first steps in the history of The Seeing Eye. They were trained by Jack Humphrey and George Eustis on the grounds of Fortunate Fields, the streets of Vevey, and hillsides of Mount Pelerin. It was a new experience for everyone involved. There was hard work, repetition, and long and tiring walks at a brisk pace. Frank experienced some bumps and bruises to his body and ego, but he was not about to be denied. (Courtesy The Seeing Eye and Emile Gos.)

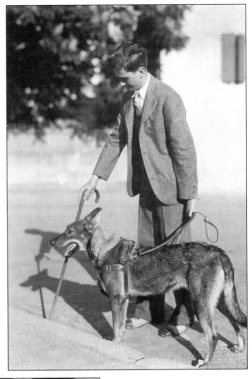

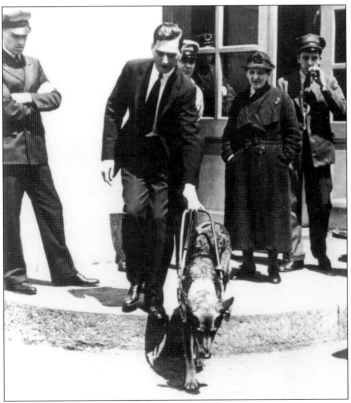

Residents of Vevey had never seen anything like this before, as Frank and Buddy negotiated the high curbs and winding streets of this quaint town on the shores of Lake Geneva. Buddy proved herself one day in training while she and her master were walking along a narrow roadway. Suddenly, a pair of runaway horses hitched to a cart galloped directly at them. Recognizing the immediate danger, Buddy pulled her master up a steep embankment and out of harm's way. Had it not been for Buddy's quick thinking, the American dog guide movement could have ended right there.

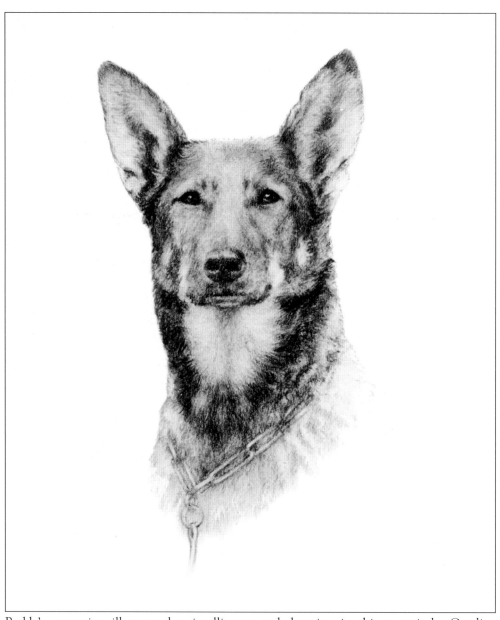

Buddy's expression illustrates her intelligence and devotion in this portrait by Caroline Thurber. The staff at Fortunate Fields selected the perfect candidate to prove to the American public that a dog could serve as the eyes of a person who could not see. Buddy demonstrated her abilities time and again, like the incident in Dayton, Ohio, when she determinedly prevented Morris Frank from falling down an open elevator shaft. She became world famous, traveling with her master across North America for years, attending speaking engagements and press conferences. Her proficiency forced the skeptics to reconsider their position and allowed The Seeing Eye to move forward. Buddy was the first of six dog guides Frank had throughout his life; all were named Buddy.

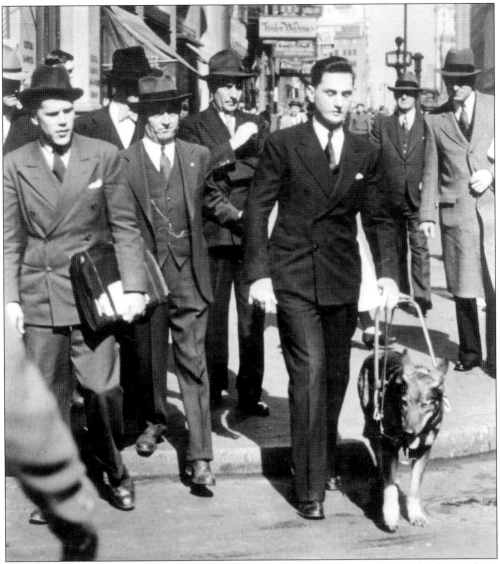

Frank and Buddy completed their training in Vevey and sailed into New York harbor on June 11, 1928. Members of the press were at the dock to greet them. One cynical newspaperman challenged Frank to cross treacherous West Street. Unaware of the extremely dangerous traffic, Frank gladly obliged. "I lost all sense of direction and surrendered myself entirely to the dog," Frank explained. "I shall never forget the next three minutes. Ten-ton trucks rocketing past, cabs blowing their horns in our ears, drivers shouting at us. When we finally made it to the other side and I realized what a really magnificent job she had done, I leaned over and gave Buddy a great big hug and told her what a good, good girl she was." The media were impressed. Frank and Buddy are shown here crossing a city street after returning to America.

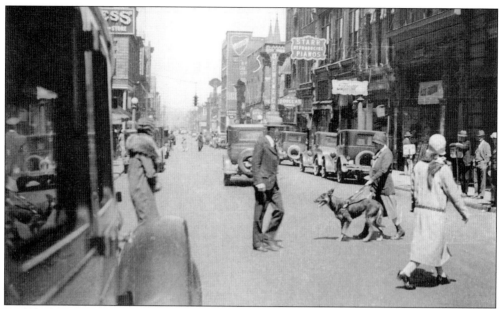

Even before Morris Frank and Buddy left Switzerland, it was decided that a dog guide school would be established in the United States. On January 29, 1929, The Seeing Eye was incorporated in Tennessee. The photographs on this and the next page show the first Seeing Eye class in training in America. They were taken in Nashville in February 1929.

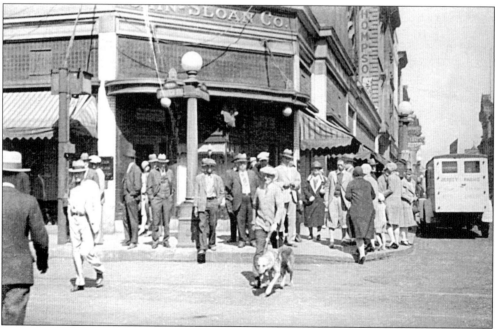

The school took its name from the headline in the *Saturday Evening Post* article. Dorothy Harrison Eustis was president, and Frank was named managing director. Fortunate Fields provided financial, supervisory, and technical support. Although at first reluctant, Jack Humphrey came to the United States to serve as the chief instructor. George Eustis might have come instead, but he and Dorothy had recently divorced.

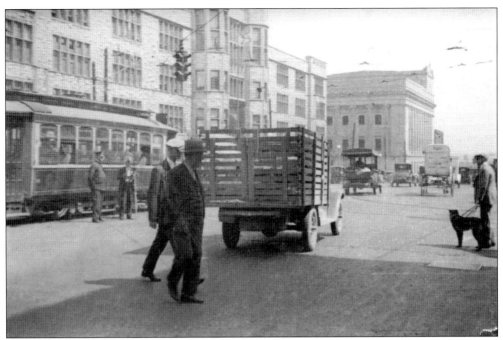

The young Morris Frank was put in charge of the day-to-day operations of the school because "he was the only one who had the guts to touch it," explained Dorothy Harrison Eustis. He had the initiative and drive necessary to get the fledgling organization up and running.

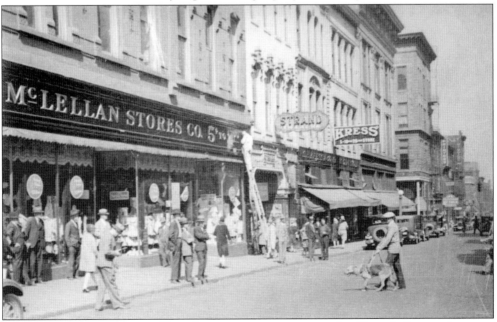

In addition to The Seeing Eye, there were two men in the United States who were experimenting with dog guides at the time: John Synikin of Minneapolis and Josef Weber, a breeder from Princeton, New Jersey. Synikin imported a shepherd from Germany in 1927 and trained it for a blind U.S. senator from Minnesota, Thomas Schall. The Seeing Eye eventually became the model for other dog guide schools that followed.

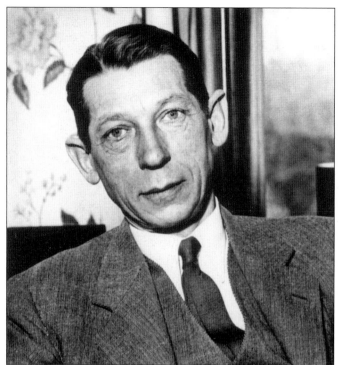

German-born Willi Ebeling lived in Dover, New Jersey, and bred German shepherds, with a special emphasis on their working abilities. After meeting Jack Humphrey, Ebeling became interested in dog guiding and wound up in Nashville, learning to become an instructor. He also supplied The Seeing Eye with some of its first dogs. Ebeling soon became the school's first administrator.

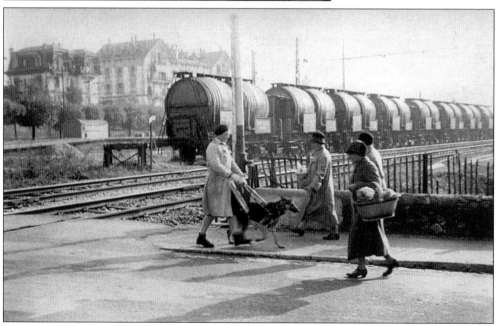

American Adelaide Clifford (shown working with a shepherd) was an original Seeing Eye instructor. While visiting in Switzerland, she became acquainted with Fortunate Fields and was soon learning the ropes with Jack Humphrey. She turned out to be a good trainer and was instrumental in the first two years of The Seeing Eye's development. Although it would be a number of years before another woman was hired as an instructor, today about half of the instructors are women.

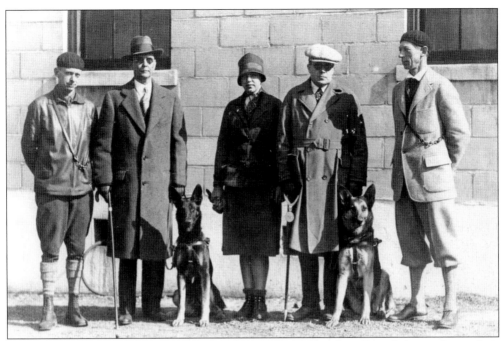

Pictured in Nashville in February 1929 is the first graduating class. From left to right are Jack Humphrey, chief instructor; Dr. Raymond Harris, student, of Savannah, Georgia, with his dog, Tartar; Adelaide Clifford, instructor; Dr. Howard Buchanan, student, of Monmouth, Illinois, with his dog, Gala; and Willi Ebeling, instructor. The photograph captures a momentous event. At that time in the United States, the general sentiment was that blind people were helpless.

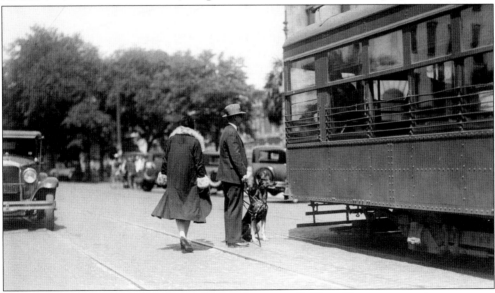

Dr. Raymond Harris and Tartar learned their lessons well. Here, Tartar stops to let a streetcar pass as the two cross Bay Street in Savannah. "Life's pathway is strewn with many pitfalls and dangers, but your dog will successfully negotiate for you all of these and protect you at all times," Harris wrote to a group of new students a month after his own graduation. (Courtesy The Seeing Eye and Foltz Studios.)

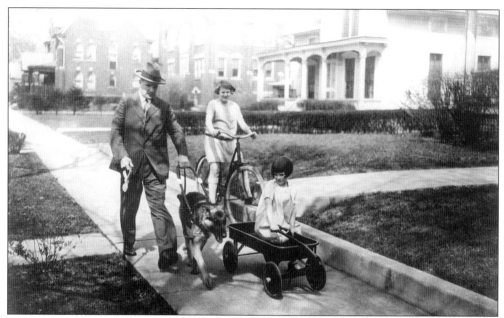

Dr. Howard Buchanan (shown with Gala skirting children at play on a sidewalk) was originally going to train in Vevey along with Morris Frank, but he became ill and had to cancel his trip. "The first day I was home, I went out with Gala alone and we went to nine different places," the doctor explained. "This is the first time since my blindness that I have been able to go when and where I pleased without asking some member of my family or a friend to go with me."

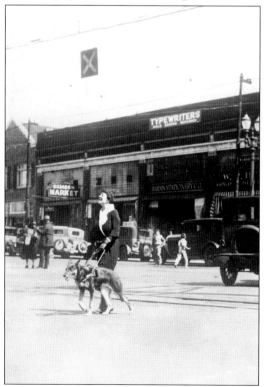

Blanche Eddy of Berkeley, California, was a student in the second class, which began on March 28, 1929. The first woman in America to have a Seeing Eye dog became a believer in the program one day during training when her dog, Beta, gently steered her around an open manhole on a congested Nashville street. Eddy was instrumental in introducing dog guides to California.

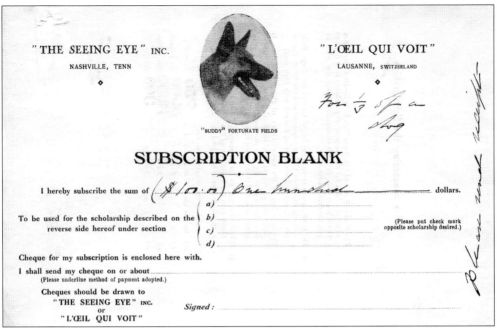

"THE SEEING EYE" INC.
NASHVILLE, TENN
◆

"BUDDY" FORTUNATE FIELDS

"L'ŒIL QUI VOIT"
LAUSANNE, SWITZERLAND
◆

SUBSCRIPTION BLANK

I hereby subscribe the sum of ($10.00) One hundred _____ dollars.

                       a) ....

To be used for the scholarship described on the   *b)* ....   (Please put check mark
reverse side hereof under section   *c)* ....   opposite scholarship desired.)

                       d) ....

Cheque for my subscription is enclosed here with.

I shall send my cheque on or about...
(Please underline method of payment adopted.)

Cheques should be drawn to
     "THE SEEING EYE" INC.   *Signed :* ....
        or
     "L'ŒIL QUI VOIT"

In the early years, students who could afford it were expected to pay for their dogs—between $170 and $375. Scholarships from individuals or groups were offered to those who did not have the means. A scholarship form is shown here. In 1934, the student fee was reduced to $150, where it remains today. The actual cost to breed, raise, and train a dog and to provide a student with a four-week training program, lodging, round-trip travel, and lifetime follow-up is now about $50,000. No one has ever been denied a Seeing Eye dog because of the inability to pay.

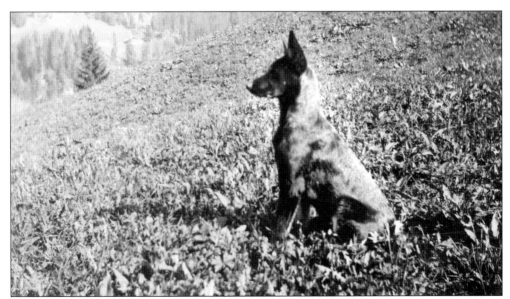

In Switzerland in 1929, Dorothy Harrison Eustis and Jack Humphrey were busy with another new school called L'Oeil qui Voit (translated as Seeing Eye). Humphrey had traveled back to Switzerland, and Ebeling handled training and administration in Nashville. Located in Lausanne, their school was established to teach European dog guide instructors.

25

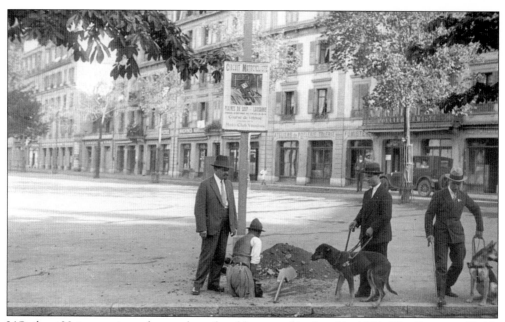

L'Oeil qui Voit experienced a number of problems, and it closed in 1934. The Fortunate Fields staff then channeled the majority of its efforts toward The Seeing Eye in the United States. This postcard shows Italian students training in Lausanne.

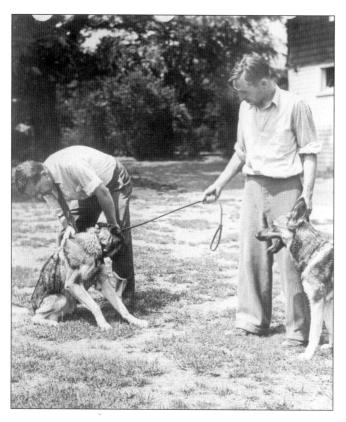

In the second half of 1929, things in Nashville became uncomfortable. It turned out that summer in the city was too long and hot for this rigorous outdoor work. Until a new headquarters was found, classes were held in different towns and cities throughout the country.

Two

AT HOME IN MORRIS COUNTY

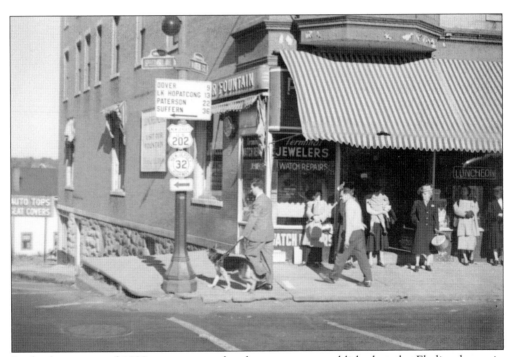

In the latter part of 1929, a temporary headquarters was established at the Ebeling home in Dover. The summer was not too hot, nor was the winter too cold. Ebeling's kennel was available for the dogs, and his home for the staff. Morristown (shown here) was located nearby. Students were housed in hotels and boardinghouses in Morristown, the seat of Morris County.

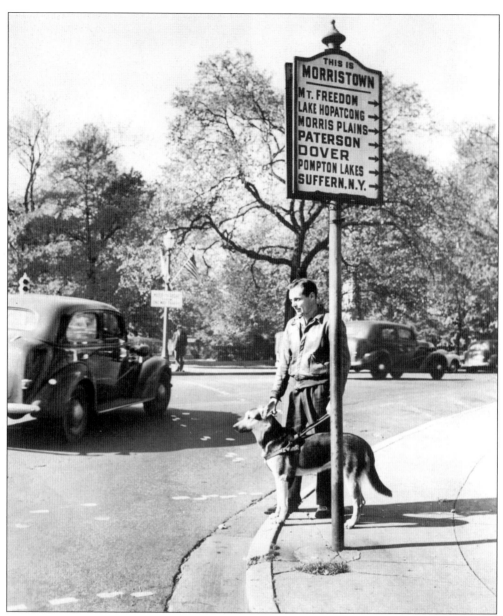

Morristown provides a diverse training site for The Seeing Eye. There are roads filled with cars, trucks, and buses; sidewalks crowded with pedestrians; traffic lights; crosswalks; quiet residential neighborhoods; an active train station; hotels; retail stores; restaurants; parks; and occasional excitement. One night, a fire broke out in a hotel where eight students were staying. They were led unscathed from the burning building by their dogs. Shown here is Ned Myrose. He started with The Seeing Eye as an apprentice instructor in 1937 and retired as director of training in 1977. Myrose supervised the training of more than 4,000 Seeing Eye dogs, including four of Morris Frank's Buddys.

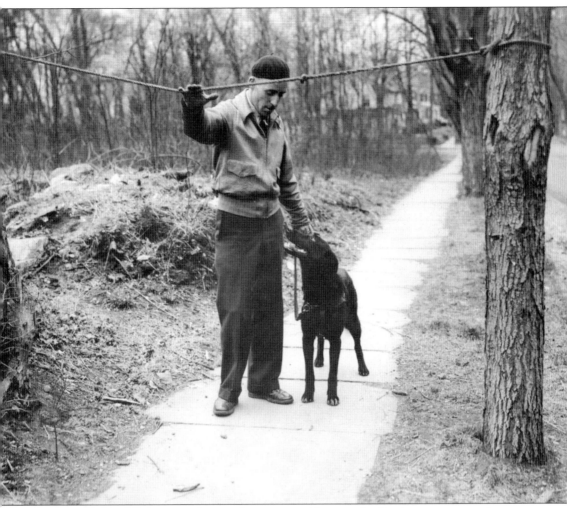

G. William "Debbie" Debetaz was born in Lausanne and became the first instructor to graduate from L'Oeil qui Voit. He joined The Seeing Eye in the United States in 1929 and stayed for 43 years. Capable instructors are a rare breed. They must be smart, physically fit, patient, steel-nerved, empathetic, able to communicate with people and dogs, and willing to work long hours (inside and outside) under all weather conditions. Today, an apprentice goes through three years of training before becoming an instructor. There is a statue of Debetaz in front of the Morris Township headquarters. Debetaz is shown teaching a dog to be aware of overhead obstructions, such as signs or tree limbs, that could endanger its master.

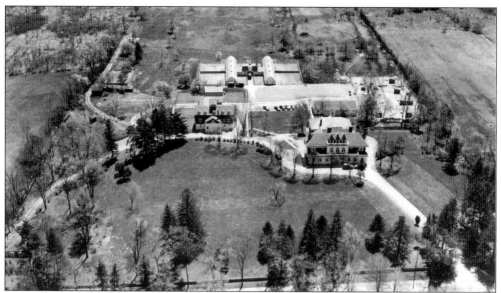

In 1931, Dorothy Harrison Eustis found a permanent home for The Seeing Eye. It was this 56-acre estate on Whippany Road in Whippany, a few miles from Morristown. "I feel we have taken a big step forward in putting The Seeing Eye on a more solid foundation," she wrote to Morris Frank after deciding on the facility. This would serve as headquarters for more than 30 years. (Courtesy The Seeing Eye and Thomas Airviews.)

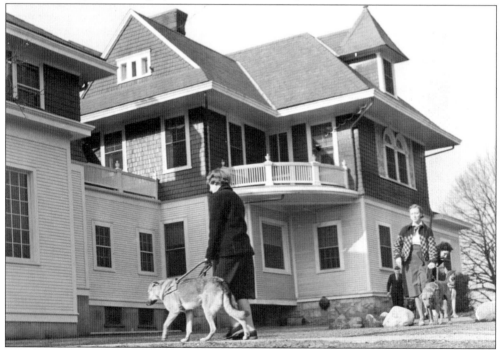

Settling into Whippany was a milestone. The Seeing Eye finally had dog training, student instruction, and student housing all on one campus, where day-to-day living situations could be practiced. The grounds were spacious, the main building was comfortable, and there was plenty of room for kennels.

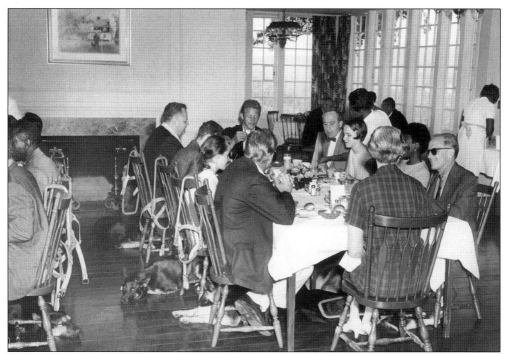

Eating meals is an important part of Seeing Eye instruction. The dining room resembles a restaurant, with each dog lying beneath the table or chair, as inconspicuous as possible. Instructors often join students at mealtimes. Students and instructors used to dress up for dinner, until the dress code was relaxed a few years ago. (Courtesy The Seeing Eye and Olson Studio.)

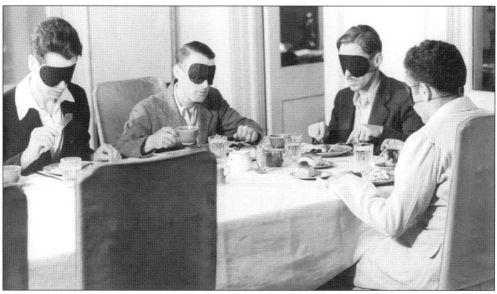

Early on, it was decided that in order for instructors to have a better understanding of what it was like to be blind, they would spend a month wearing a blindfold—day and night—as part of their education. Today, they are under blindfold for one week. They go through the same training as do students and emerge as more empathetic instructors.

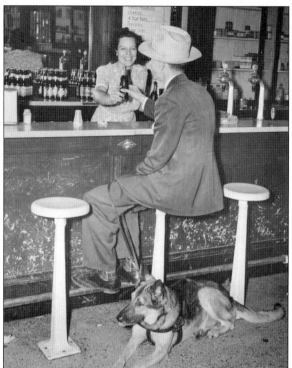

Not every public eatery was as welcoming as this one in 1941, when Floyd Sparleman stopped for a beverage with his dog, Flocke. Many restaurants, hotels, and retailers did not allow dogs in their establishments—be they dog guides or not. (Courtesy The Seeing Eye and the Dallas Morning News.)

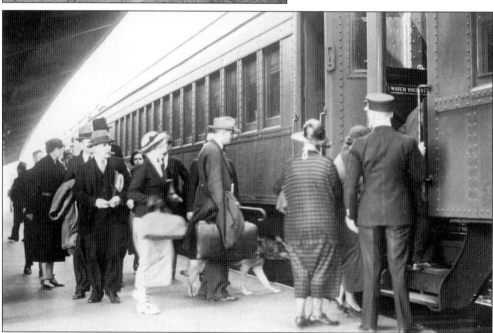

Trains often relegated Seeing Eye dogs to the baggage car, despite the difficulties incurred by their masters. The Pennsylvania Railroad became the first to allow Seeing Eye dogs to ride as passengers along with their companions, after some convincing by Dorothy Harrison Eustis. "Solutions to the challenges of blindness begin with the individual but can be enhanced by the support of family and friends, as well as society at large," according to The Seeing Eye.

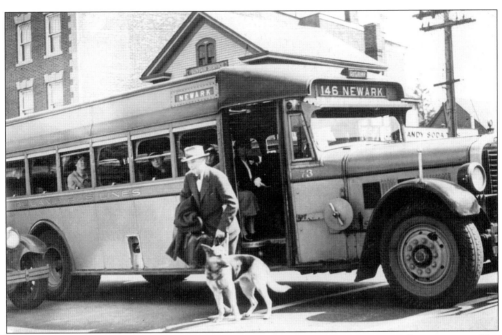

The Seeing Eye spent many years fighting the powers that be to gain equal access to public transportation and facilities for dog guides. In 1992, the Americans with Disabilities Act became the law of the land, prohibiting discrimination against a blind person with a dog guide. All states and Canadian provinces have similar laws.

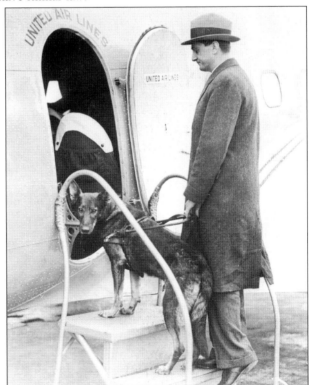

This was a poignant moment in Seeing Eye history. It was Buddy's last trip, after crossing the country for years with Morris Frank, spreading the word about The Seeing Eye. The companions had just convinced United Airlines to allow dog guides to fly together with their masters. Buddy died from cancer in 1938, soon after this photograph was taken.

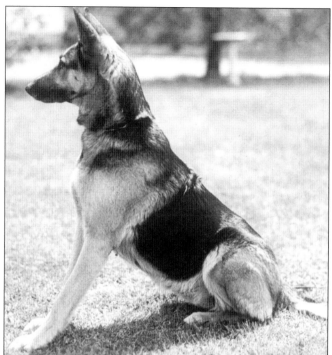

The characteristics Jack Humphrey looked for in a dog were intelligence, a willingness to learn, strength and stamina, good health, average size, not shy, not startled by sudden noises, aggressive enough to lead its master where necessary but not overly aggressive, and an average sense of smell. An example of a dog with the right stuff was Kara (shown here), who belonged to Mervyn Sinclair, former president of the Pennsylvania Council for the Blind.

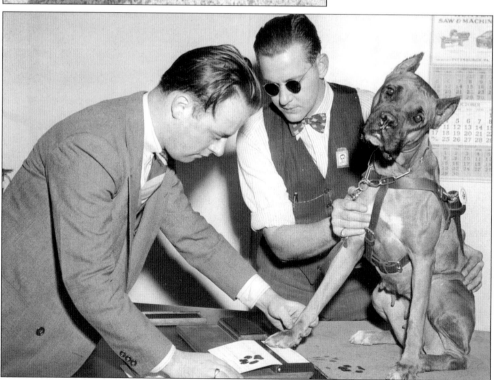

Although German shepherds were recruited most often in the early days, The Seeing Eye has successfully trained several dozen breeds over the years. Shown here is Duchess being paw-printed so that she can accompany her master to his defense job during World War II.

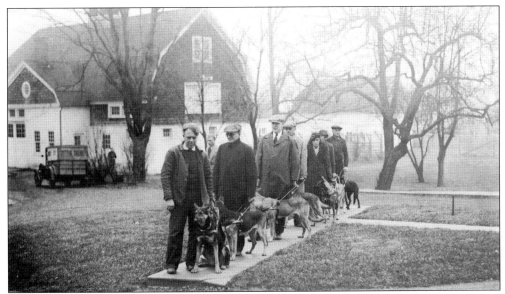

The Great Depression impacted the school in the 1930s. Dorothy Harrison Eustis and several friends kept it afloat, but additional resources were needed. Eustis embarked on a fund-raising campaign that eventually led to financial solvency. The Seeing Eye is a philanthropy that is supported by contributions, trust income, bequests, and endowment earnings. It has never accepted government aid of any kind.

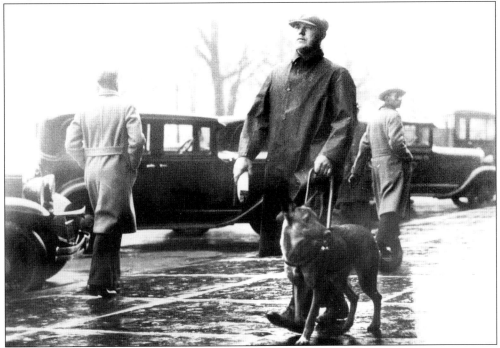

Students must be at least 16 years old and in good health. They have come from all walks of life, and the common thread among them is a strong desire to reach a new level of independence. One to two percent of people who are legally blind choose to team up with a dog guide.

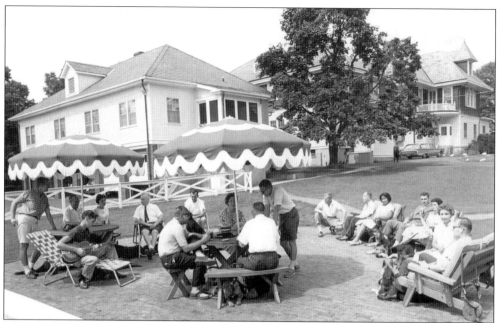

Although students are made to feel comfortable, as can be seen on the patio of the Whippany campus, The Seeing Eye's philosophy was to avoid coddling them. Morris Frank learned this lesson in Vevey. On his first solo walk with Buddy, Frank wound up with a few jarring bumps, as Jack Humphrey looked on from afar. Frank was angry. "When you go back to the United States, I won't be there," Humphrey told his student. "Your future's up to you." Frank later agreed.

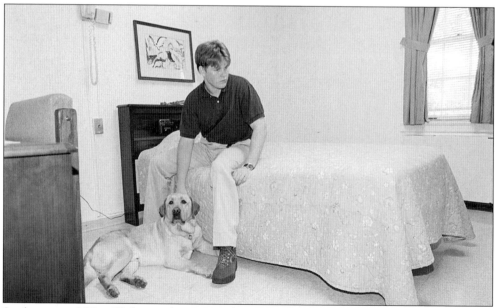

Students spend 20 to 27 days at the campus, learning the techniques required to work as a team with their dog. It is a pleasant, homelike atmosphere. By 1938, there were not enough bedrooms in the main house, so male students were moved to another building on the campus. The student residence today has 24 private rooms, each with private bath.

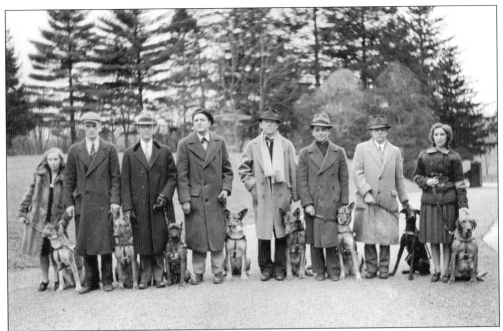

Eleven students graduated from The Seeing Eye in 1931; the number grew to 144 in 1940. By 1950, the total reached 187. Eight students were assigned to each class. Today, approximately 300 people from the United States and Canada come to The Seeing Eye each year—new students as well as those returning for a successor dog. The fee for a successor dog is $50.

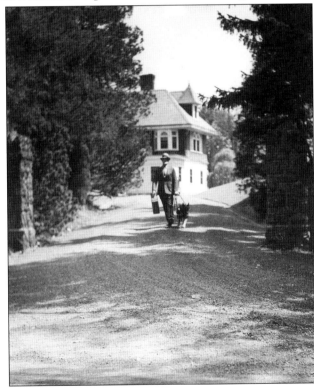

Much had changed by 1963. Dorothy Harrison Eustis and Willi Ebeling had passed away; Jack Humphrey and Morris Frank were retired. The Seeing Eye had outgrown the Whippany facility. It was time to move on.

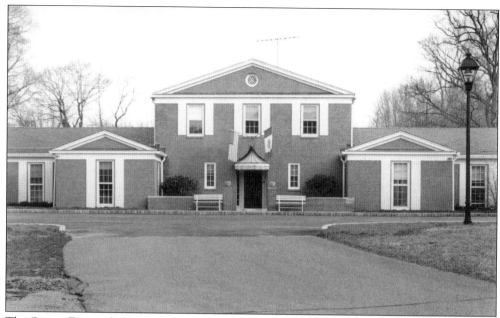

The Seeing Eye settled in its present Morris Township location in 1965. The brick Georgian-style main building houses a student wing with 24 private rooms, a dining room, a lounge, an exercise room, a library and technology center, a laundry room, administrative offices, and a gracious entrance hall. It sits atop 60 acres of lush green lawns dotted with grand old trees and looks out over the Washington Valley. A half-mile pathway winds along the grounds, allowing students to practice with their dogs. The milieu is reminiscent of a gracious estate. (Above courtesy The Seeing Eye and E. James Pitrone.)

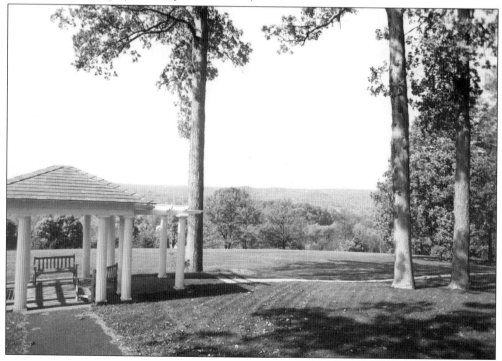

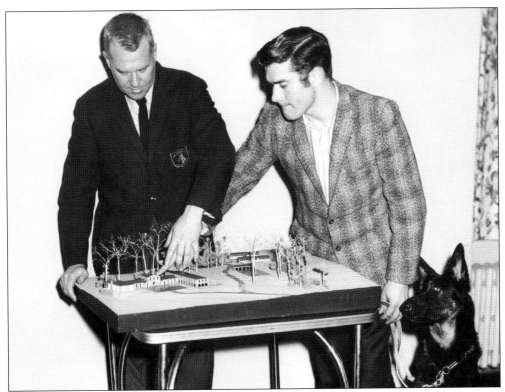

Scale models with Braille labels were designed to help students learn their way around campus. In this view, instructor Dick Krokus gives a student a feel for the exterior. Another model of The Seeing Eye teaches students the indoor layout. The Seeing Eye believes in a personalized approach to learning. (Courtesy The Seeing Eye and Dahlmeyer Studios.)

A relief map of Morristown allows students to learn the streets where they will practice. In an unfamiliar location, a blind person asks for directions, the same as a sighted person. Dogs are trained to obey commands, but it is up to the master to let the dog know which way to go.

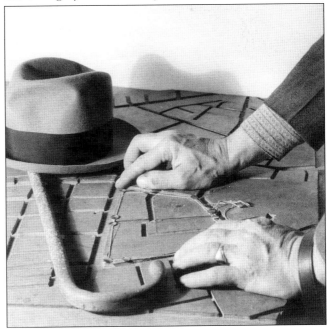

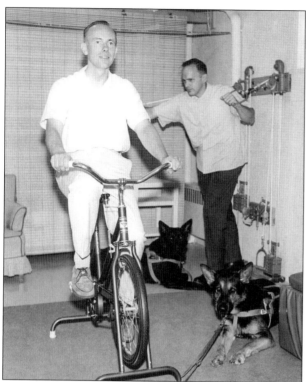

Students must be in good physical condition before they are accepted into the program. Training requires lots of walking each day. After they graduate, students are expected to walk their dogs daily to keep them fit. Two healthy students are shown working out in the exercise room with their dogs at their feet. (Courtesy The Seeing Eye and Dahlmeyer Studios.)

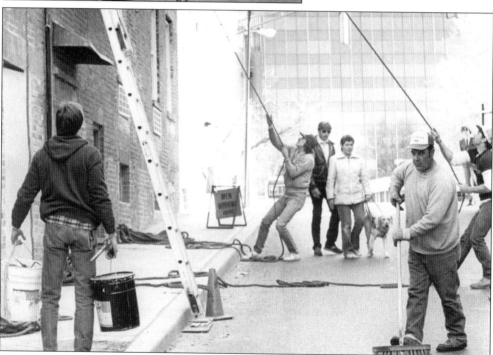

This is an example of why keeping fit has always been considered important. Students head outdoors in all types of weather and must be prepared for whatever comes across their path. (Courtesy The Seeing Eye and E. James Pitrone.)

40

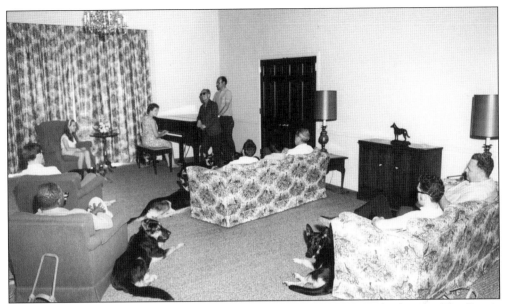

After a hard day's work, students and their dogs often take it easy in the lounge. The Seeing Eye can accommodate 24 students at the same time. While the majority of program costs are underwritten by charitable contributions, students are assessed a small fee, $150 for their first dog and $50 for each successor dog. The Seeing Eye has always believed that students maintain greater self-respect when they assume a portion of their obligation. (Courtesy The Seeing Eye and Olson Studio.)

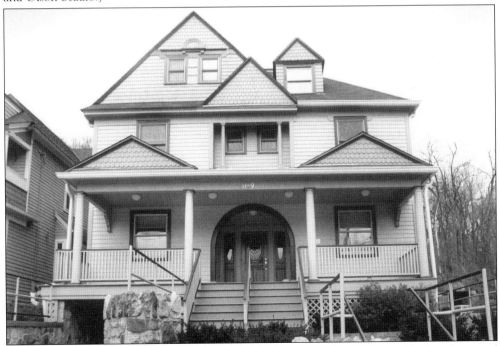

The Mount Kemble Center in Morristown was purchased in the 1980s to afford students and instructors a place to train as well as a spot to rest and regroup during downtown training exercises. (Courtesy The Seeing Eye and E. James Pitrone.)

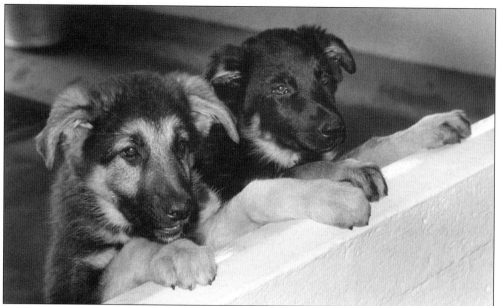

Good breeding has been the cornerstone of the program from the beginning. Jack Humphrey took a scientific approach. First, he determined the mental and physical characteristics required for the ideal dog guide, and then Fortunate Fields began breeding for those qualities. The Seeing Eye's breeding program has improved the dogs genetically over successive generations. (Courtesy The Seeing Eye and E. James Pitrone.)

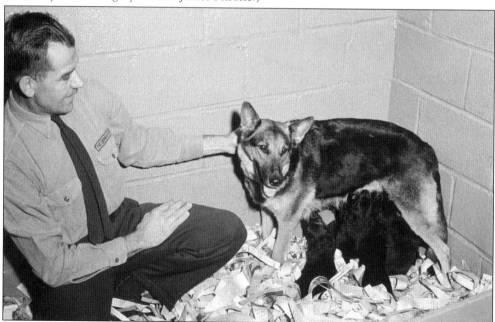

Humphrey maintained that inbreeding had eliminated the working qualities of German shepherds. He endeavored to correct this by breeding dogs that were only distantly related. Today, males are mated 15 times. Females are bred until they are 48 months old. The mother's love and discipline in the early weeks of a puppy's life are very important in the development process. (Courtesy The Seeing Eye and J. Stanley Brandt.)

42

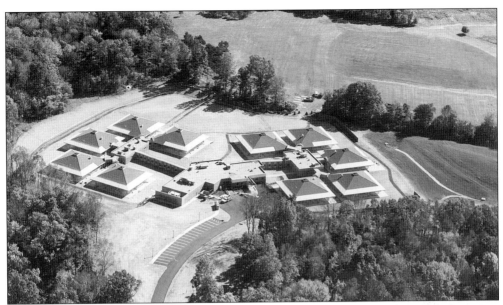

The Seeing Eye began breeding shepherds in 1941 at Whippany. Until then, dogs were obtained from Fortunate Fields, Ebeling's kennel, and other breeders. The breeding operation moved to a more spacious farm in Mendham, New Jersey, in 1948. More than 10,000 puppies were born in Mendham. A new state-of-the-art canine reproduction and maternity center (above) was opened in Chester, New Jersey, in 2001. The 62,500-square-foot facility is located on 330 acres of land. The Seeing Eye Breeding Station at Chester houses 90 dogs, excluding puppies, and supports the whelping of 100 litters annually. The Seeing Eye's breeding program is recognized as one of the most sophisticated in the world. Members of The Seeing Eye board of trustees and staff are shown below with the guest speaker during the ribbon-cutting ceremony in Chester.

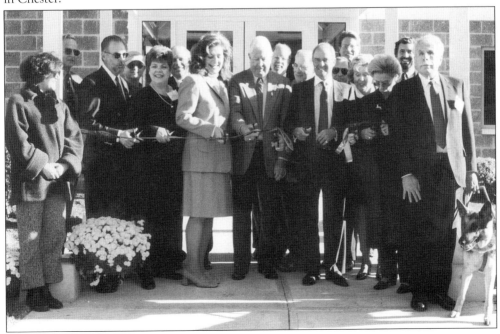

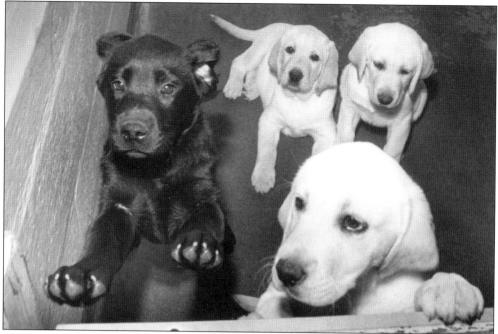

The Seeing Eye began breeding Labradors for the first time in 1979. Golden retrievers are also bred, as well as a golden-lab mix. Although as many as 90 percent of the dogs-in-training come from the breeding station, some are still obtained from outside sources. (Courtesy The Seeing Eye and E. James Pitrone.)

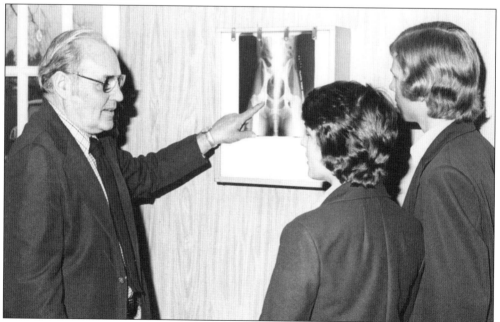

Breeding for healthy hips has been of paramount importance. Hip dysplasia eliminated many dogs that would have otherwise been good candidates for guiding. By 1994, The Seeing Eye had reduced hip dysplasia in German shepherds from 30 percent to five percent, and in Labrador retrievers from 18 percent to nearly zero.

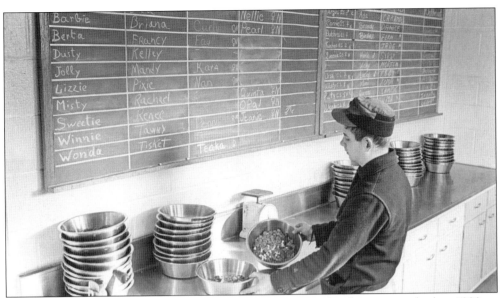

Jack Humphrey began keeping meticulous records on puppy development in the late 1920s, a practice that remains in effect today. When they are about eight weeks old, puppies are sent to live with volunteers who raise them until they are about 18 months old. The best Seeing Eye dogs are well bred and cared for, socialized, trained, and motivated by a desire to please.

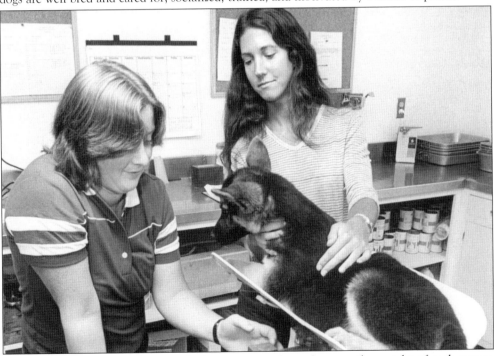

In addition to measuring how much they eat, records are kept on the weight of each puppy. Laboratory technicians at the breeding station are shown weighing in this young shepherd. Puppies that are not accepted into the program are adopted by loving families. Retired dog guides that do not stay with the master or with the master's friends or relatives are taken back by The Seeing Eye and are also adopted. (Courtesy The Seeing Eye and E. James Pitrone.)

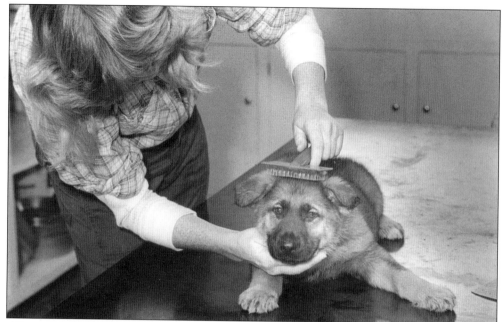

All puppies are groomed regularly, an important component in health management. Students must groom their dogs daily during training and are expected to keep up the practice once they graduate. (Courtesy The Seeing Eye and E. James Pitrone.)

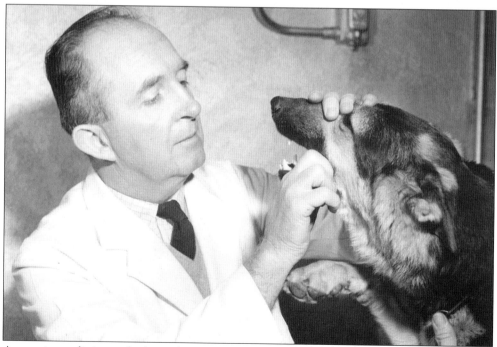

A veterinary clinic was built on the campus in 1979. At first, there were no veterinarians on staff, so local practitioners like this one held regular office hours at the clinic. In 1991, a full-time veterinarian was hired. Today, there are three on staff to consult with graduates and to tend to the puppies, breeders, and dogs-in-training. (Courtesy The Seeing Eye and Hugelmeyer.)

Dolores Holle, VMD, director of canine health management, and her staff oversee the Vincent A. Stabile Canine Health Center, which opened at the Washington Valley campus in 1997. The center provides ongoing care for as many as 300 dogs that are on campus at any given time. Dr. Holle is shown here examining a young Labrador retriever.

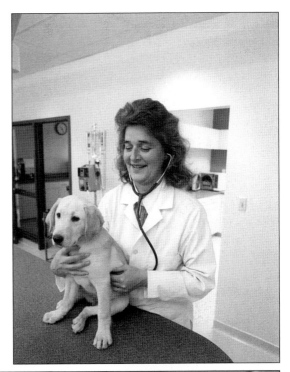

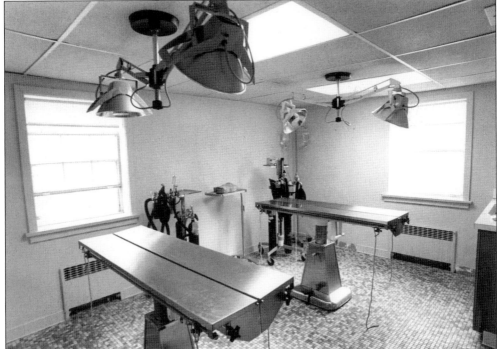

The health center originally included an operating room, recovery room, an x-ray room, and a holding pen. The Seeing Eye infrastructure had come a long way since the early days in Nashville, where Morris Frank rented a small office for the new corporation, and one of the first two students lodged at the YMCA. (Courtesy The Seeing Eye and E. James Pitrone.)

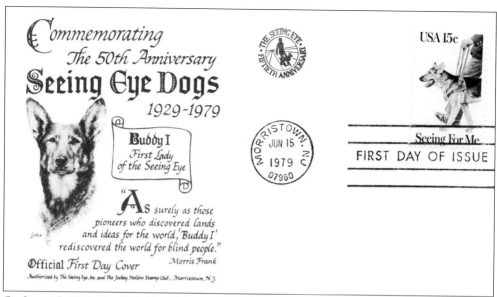

Commemorating
The 50th Anniversary
Seeing Eye Dogs
1929-1979

Buddy I
First Lady
of the Seeing Eye

"**A**S surely as those
pioneers who discovered lands
and ideas for the world, 'Buddy I'
rediscovered the world for blind people."
Morris Frank

Official *First Day Cover*
Authorized by The Seeing Eye, Inc. and The Jockey Hollow Stamp Club, Morristown, N.J.

MORRISTOWN. N.J.
JUN 15
1979
07960

USA 15c

Seeing For Me
FIRST DAY OF ISSUE

On June 15, 1979, the U.S. Postal Service issued a 15¢ commemorative stamp, recognizing the service performed by dog guides on the 50th anniversary of The Seeing Eye. "They [Seeing Eye graduates] and their dogs have proved the wisdom of Mrs. Eustis' vision and the soundness of the training developed by Jack Humphrey and others, and they have justified the faith and courage of Morris S. Frank," said the postal service.

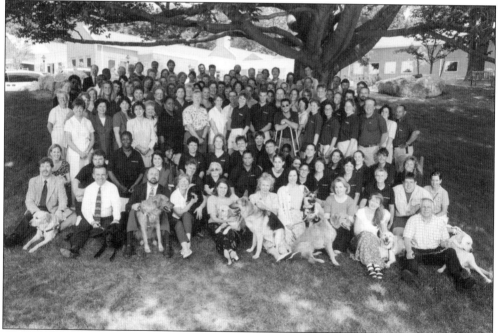

From a small group of pioneers in 1929, the staff of The Seeing Eye grew to 170 in 2001. In addition, scores of volunteers assist the organization in a variety of ways. This staff photograph was taken on the campus grounds in 1999. Other dog guide schools operate throughout the country. The Seeing Eye is the oldest school in North America and has set the standard for others throughout the world to follow.

Three
CHALLENGES, GREAT
AND SMALL

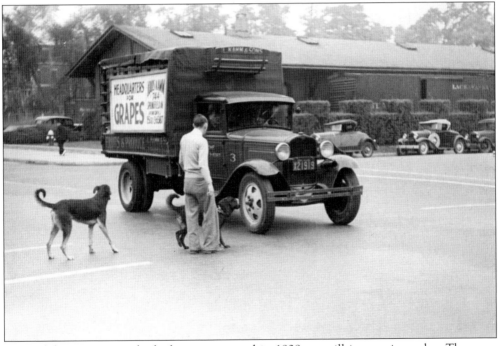

Most of the training methods that were started in 1929 are still in practice today. There are several categories of instruction: training apprentices to become instructors, training young dogs to become guides, and training people who are blind or visually impaired to work as a team with their dogs. The dog guide pictured here is learning to deal with distractions, including the curious canine at its heels.

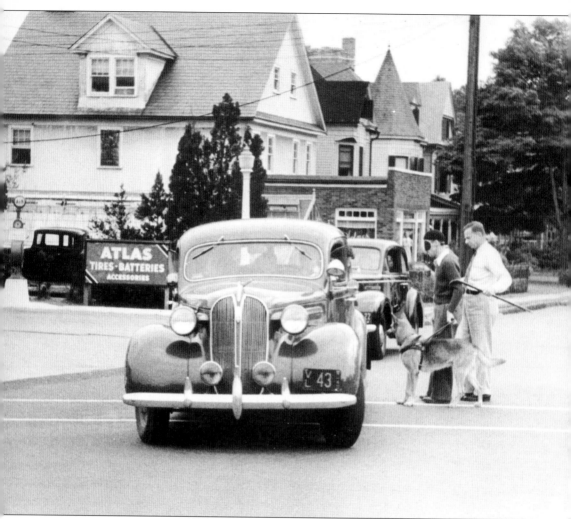

Instructor G. William Debetaz (left) and Jack Humphrey are shown walking through a training exercise. Finding capable instructors has been a major challenge since 1929. Apprentices go through three years of training. Once it is completed, they find that the workdays are long and hard, sometimes as many as 13 hours per day. It is a physically demanding job—instructors can walk up to 15 miles each day in all types of weather. Intelligence and character are required. The ability to get things done is essential, as is the spirit to overcome discouragement. At various times, there have been salary issues. At first, Dorothy Harrison Eustis and Humphrey believed they could find experienced dog trainers and teach them to be good dog guide instructors. Generally, that did not work. The Fortunate Fields methodologies were very specific and not always compatible with other types of training. In the first 12 years of existence, The Seeing Eye produced just six instructors.

Apprentice instructors spend their first several months as kennel assistants, working, observing, and learning about the dogs. After a time, they move on to initial obedience training and then receive dogs of their own to train. It takes four months to train a dog. (Courtesy The Seeing Eye and the Equity Press.)

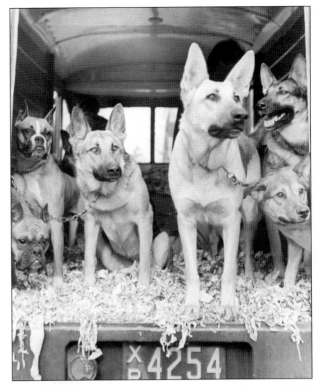

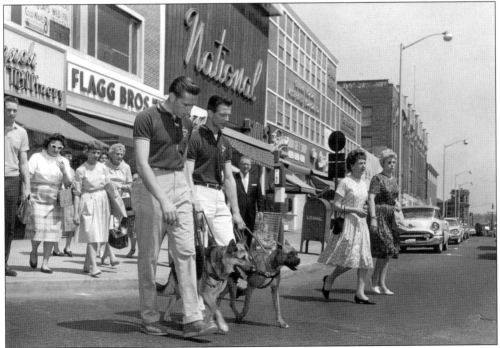

Tact is an important quality an instructor must possess; it is instinctive, something that cannot be taught. Instructors have to be friendly yet firm as they work with students and the dogs. (Courtesy The Seeing Eye and Rue Studio.)

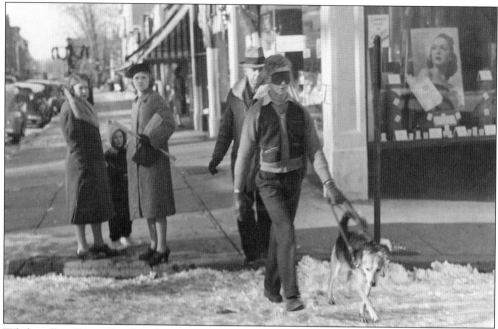

While still in Switzerland, Jack Humphrey recognized a problem: sometimes a sighted instructor would inadvertently give small physical cues to a dog, such as a hand or arm movement, at the same time he issued a voice command. Some dogs responded to the physical signal instead of the verbal. After that discovery, a mandatory traffic test with the instructor blindfolded was established before a dog was graduated. (Courtesy The Seeing Eye and H.C. Dorer.)

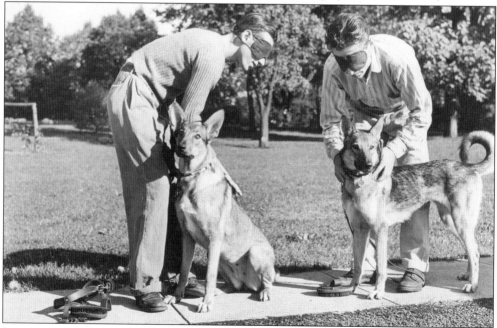

Instructors must learn to hook up the dog's harness without the advantage of sight. In turn, they teach this skill to their students. It becomes an important daily activity for students and graduates. (Courtesy The Seeing Eye and Sam Shere, International News Photos.)

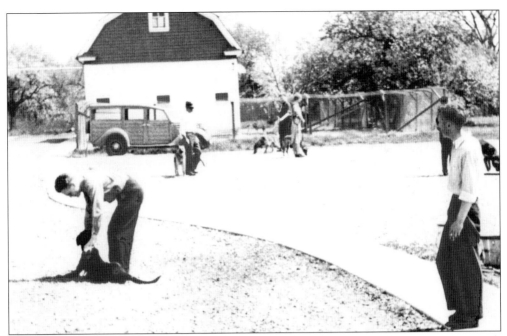

Instructors begin their day by feeding their dogs breakfast at the kennel and then playing with them for a while. After that, the dogs-in-training begin their lessons. Each instructor is responsible for training eight to 10 dogs at a time. This photograph was taken at the Whippany campus.

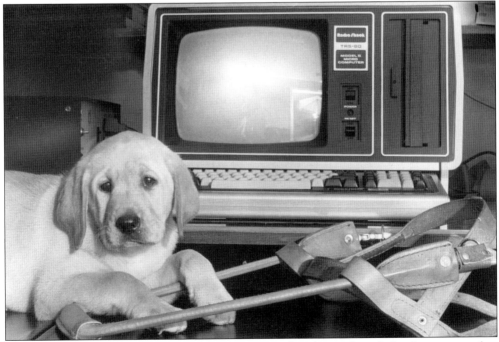

Although many dogs are smart enough to become guides, those selected also demonstrate that they are responsive to instruction—they are teachable. Computer proficiency is not required, but the dogs must want to learn and then to put their education into practice. (Courtesy The Seeing Eye and E. James Pitrone.)

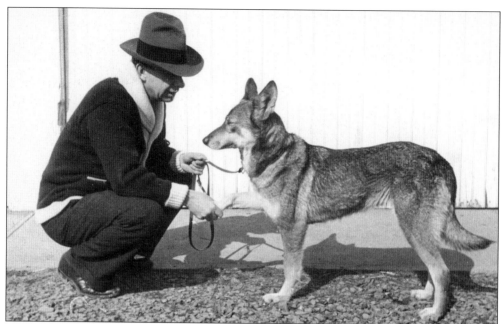

By nature, dogs like to please humans. At The Seeing Eye, they are rewarded by a pat on the head and verbal praise when they obey. When they disobey, they are told "pfui," which is a German expression meaning "shame on you" that Jack Humphrey (shown here) started using at Fortunate Fields. They are also corrected by a tug on the leash.

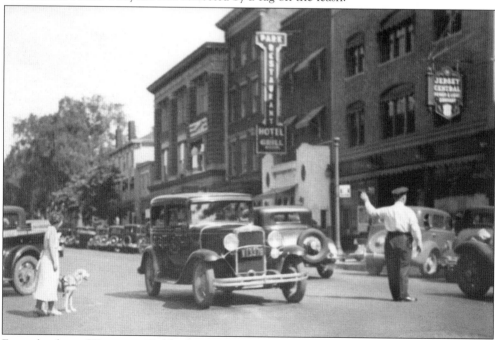

From the days of Fortunate Fields, dog guide education has been different than other training methods, which teach command and obey. Seeing Eye dogs were taught to "command and obey if it is okay." This is the difference between training a dog and educating a dog. Seeing Eye dogs make life-and-death decisions.

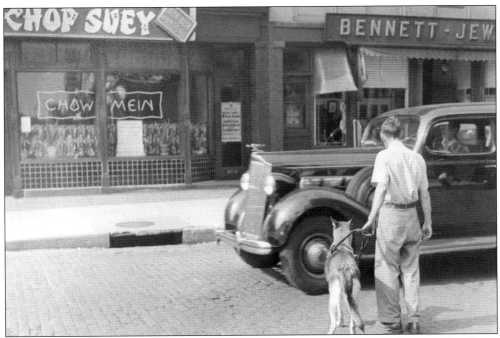

The most important lesson a Seeing Eye dog learns is "intelligent disobedience." The dog is taught to judge a situation and disobey a command if it puts its master into danger. Although instructor Curtis Weeman is telling the dog to go forward, it intelligently stops to prevent them both from being run over.

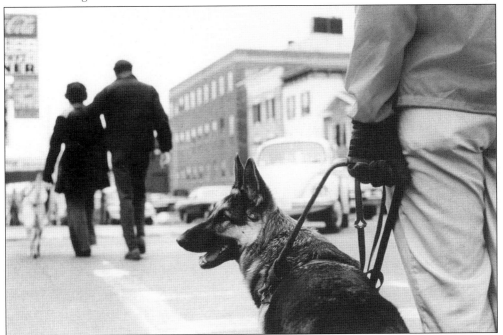

To achieve this level of intelligence, Jack Humphrey believed that the instructor must understand the dog and its point of view. If a dog could learn to comprehend what its master wanted, the dog's ability to learn was almost unlimited, Humphrey reasoned.

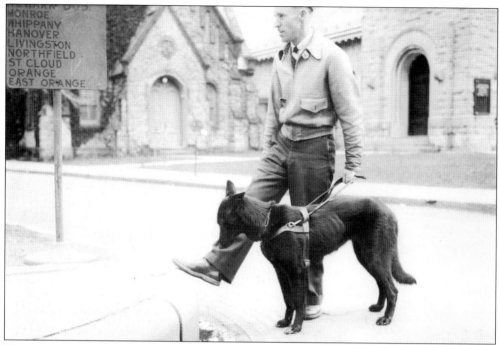

Years ago, G. William Debetaz taught this shepherd to stop when they reached the curb in Morristown so that the instructor could feel where to place his foot. This method has been updated because of heavier and faster traffic. Today, dogs learn "touch and go," a process in which the dog pauses slightly at the curb and then continues. This allows the pair to get out of the street faster.

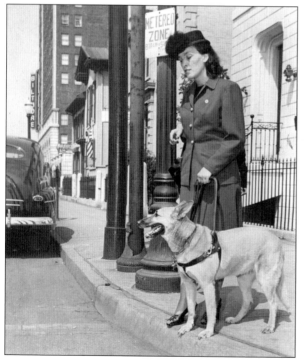

Rounded curbs have posed a problem as far back as Vevey. When a dog comes to the end of a block, it guides its master to the curb directly ahead and stops. The blind person then gives the command to go right, left, or forward, and the dog proceeds straight to the opposite curb. If the curb does not have sharply defined corners, the dog can become confused on which direction to face and may cross in the wrong direction. That is not the case, however, in this photograph.

A dog must learn to stop when it reaches a stairway in order for its master to get his footing. The combination of the dog's pull and the angle of a staircase can be tricky at first for the new student. In addition to the stairs to consider, the retriever shown here guides its master confidently through a crowded parking lot. (Courtesy The Seeing Eye and E. James Pitrone.)

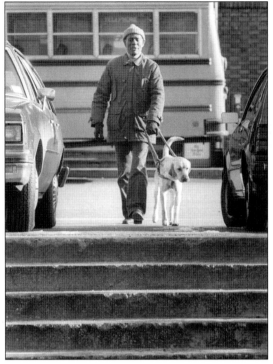

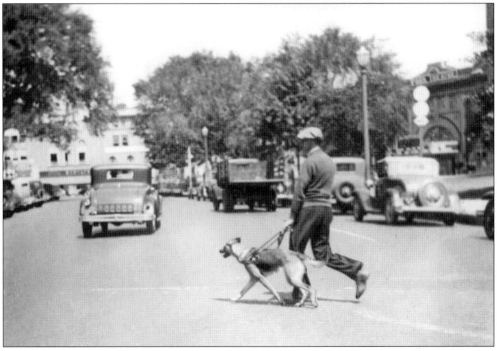

This 1930s photograph shows a shepherd obeying its master's instruction. The commands that a dog guide learns today include *sit*, *heel*, *come*, *forward*, *right*, and *left*. Dogs must learn to respond promptly to the commands of its master. Some dogs do not possess the concentration or confidence needed to be a guide and are removed from the program to be adopted.

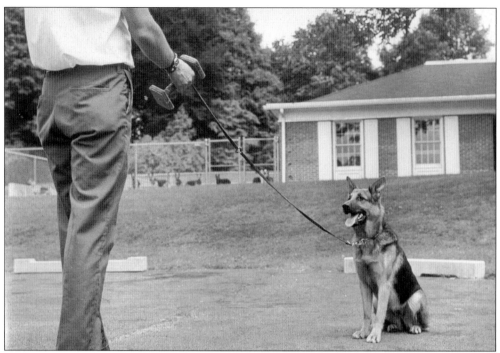

As its kennel mates look on, this shepherd-in-training obeys instructor Gary Mattoon. The Seeing Eye uses a system of affectionate rewards and gentle corrections to teach the dogs obedience. Corporal punishment is not used. It takes about 16 weeks of repetition, praise, and correction before a dog is ready to meet its new master.

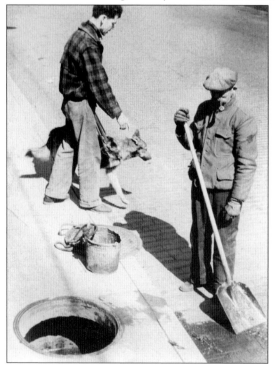

Some breeds are very smart but do not necessarily make good dog guides. For example, they may not possess the initiative or responsibility to avoid an open manhole. That could have been a problem here.

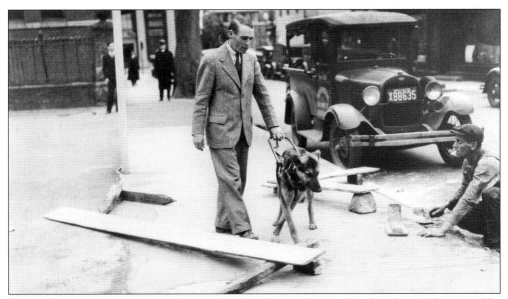

The ability to reason separates Seeing Eye dogs from others and makes dog guiding possible. Although it is supposed to proceed directly forward, the shepherd in this 1930s photograph reasons that it must go around the obstruction for the safety of its master. Instructors teach this by setting up obstacles, telling the dog to go forward, bumping into the obstruction, and then showing the dog that it should have gone around.

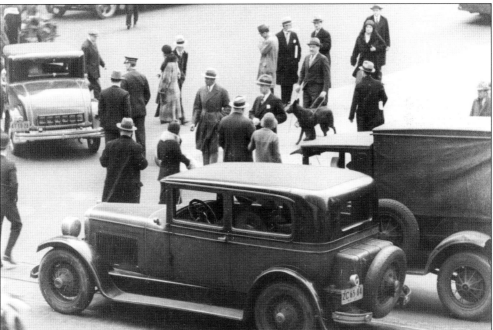

Dogs that are frightened by loud noises are rejected. Jack Humphrey tested his dogs for what he called "gun-sureness" by setting off fireworks near the animals. Sudden noises, such as the backfiring of a car, can be a danger to the blind person if the dog is shy of loud noises. Many dogs who are otherwise qualified have failed for this reason. This street scene in the 1930s surely has its share of unexpected sounds.

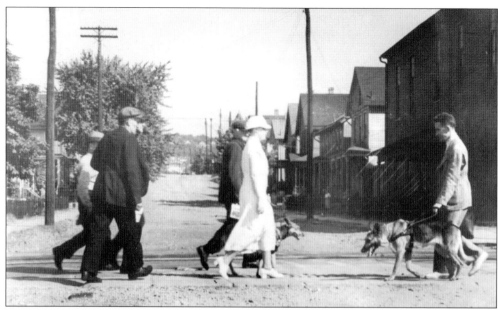

At Fortunate Fields, Humphrey realized that apprentice instructors were not always conveying their verbal messages to the dogs clearly and with the right tone, so he devised a lesson in voice culture. He taught them to direct their voices at a point between a dog's ears, as if speaking right to its brain. He also standardized the tone of the commands. The technique worked. The instructors and students shown c. 1937 in Wilkes Barre, Pennsylvania, communicated properly with their dogs.

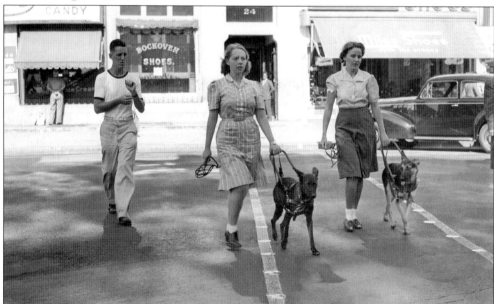

Dogs are taught to walk on the left side of their masters, with a little more than half the body of the dog ahead of the person, as shown in this photograph in Morristown. "The dog always works on your left side, between you and the pedestrian traffic," Jack Humphrey told Morris Frank the first day of his training. (Courtesy The Seeing Eye and Sam Shere, International News Photos.)

At an intersection, a master will listen for the flow of the traffic before telling his dog to go forward. Dog guides are not taught to pay attention to traffic lights. The right-turn-on-red law has caused more than one near miss for people who are blind. Instructor Howard Kane is shown giving a lesson in Morristown. (Courtesy The Seeing Eye and Rue Studio.)

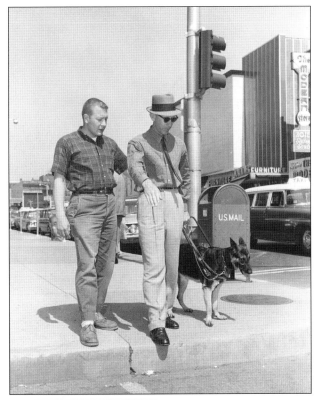

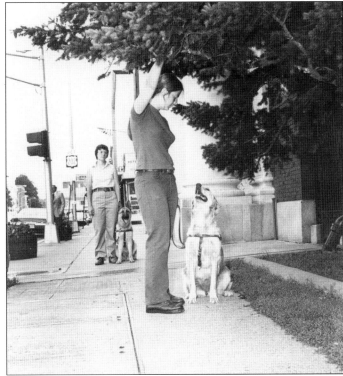

Another important skill a Seeing Eye dog learns is the ability to prevent its master from bumping into objects that are over the dog's head but not the master's. Dogs that have perfected this feat do not even seem to look up when they steer their companions around signs, awnings, and so on. Instructor Kathy Waite is shown teaching her dog to avoid a tree limb. (Courtesy The Seeing Eye and Micky Fox.)

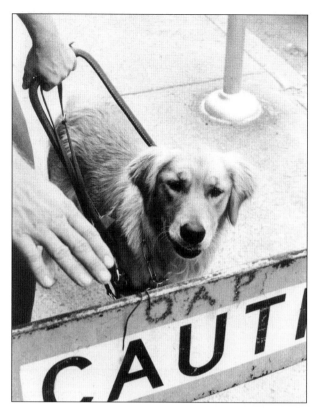

The first harness with a semirigid, U-shaped handle was used in the early 1930s. The device communicates the dog's movements to its master. It is strapped around the dog's chest and shoulders in a way that does not restrict movement. A leash is attached that enables the person to remain connected even if the handle is dropped. The leash is also used to correct the dog if a mistake is made.

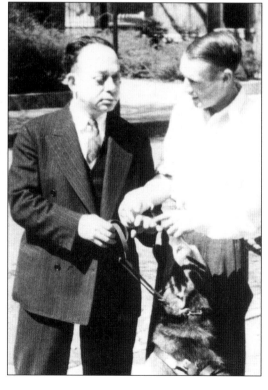

This student is learning the proper use of the harness in Whippany. It takes practice to get it on and off the dog, especially for people who cannot see. Morris Frank found this out the first few times he tried, accidentally poking Buddy in the eye, pinching her ear, and catching the chest strap on her nose. Frank and other early students also walked with a cane in their right hand, although this practice was soon eliminated.

Before students are accepted into the program, they must be proficient in the use of the white cane. The cane is used for orientation and mobility by swinging it from side to side to make sure there is safe clearance before taking a step. (Courtesy The Seeing Eye and the Office of the Superintendent of Schools of Alameda County.)

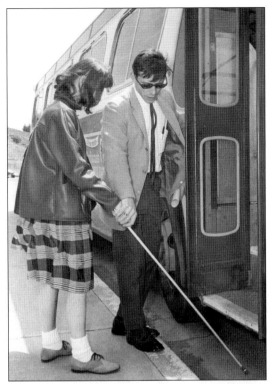

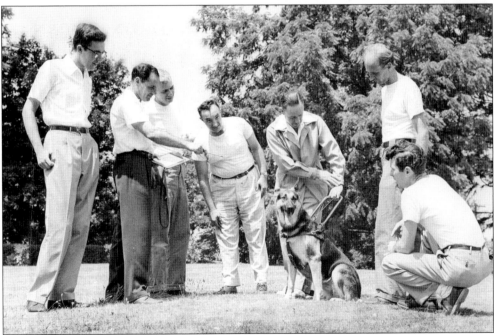

Seeing Eye dogs are taught to work together as a team with their master to create an effective working partnership. The dog sees and avoids obstacles and other dangers, but it is the person who commands and directs the dog and who must know their location, destination, and route. These instructors in Whippany are recording a German shepherd's progress.

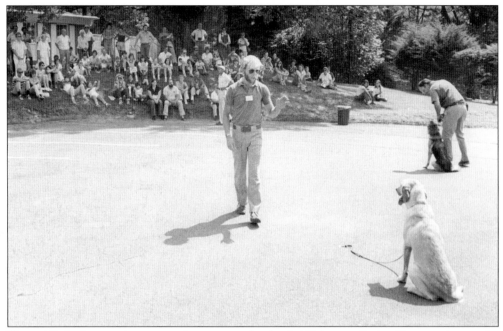

The public looks on as instructors demonstrate the dogs' abilities at a Seeing Eye open house. An instructor recruitment booklet published in 1938 discussed some of the job benefits: "It is the reward of achievement—the reward of molding raw and sometimes doubtful material into a finished product and knowing that it is good. Probably no men in America can do this more often or more thoroughly than Seeing Eye instructors." (Courtesy The Seeing Eye and E. James Pitrone.)

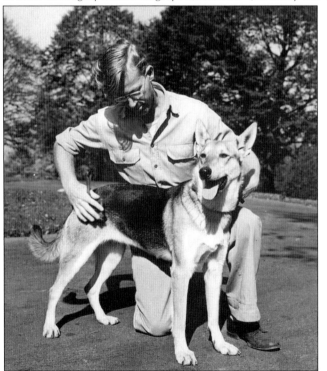

During the months they are together, instructors form a bond with their dogs-in-training. They spend quite a bit of time together, and there is mutual affection. As a result of this friendship, it generally takes a short while for dogs to unite with their new masters. Instructor John McDevitt is shown with Daisy during her daily grooming in 1946.

This instructor and student are practicing the Juno walk, one of the first things a student learns. The instructor holds the harness, and the student holds the U-shaped handle as they walk and practice. In addition to giving the student a feel for what is to come, the Juno walk allows the instructor to observe the student, which helps to match the appropriate dog with the student's physical abilities and lifestyle. (Courtesy The Seeing Eye and Micky Fox.)

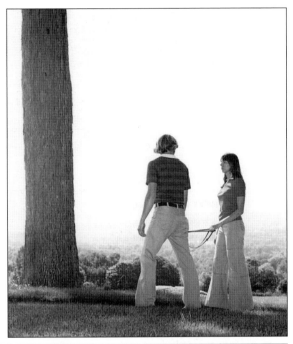

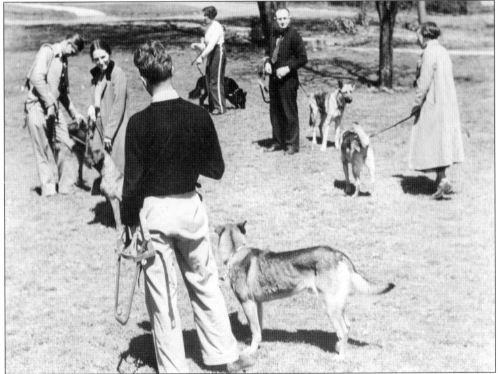

Not every master and dog turn out to be a good match, but these students in Whippany look like they are getting along just fine with their new companions. Dogs, like people, have distinct personalities, and sometimes the chemistry does not work. If this occurs, in training or after graduation, a new dog will be provided.

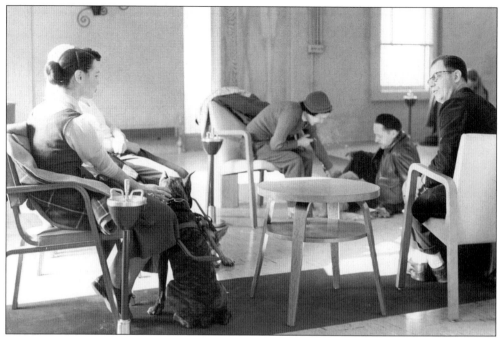

Students meet their new companions for the first time on a Monday. The dogs have completed their education, and the student training phase begins. At school, the students and dogs are together 24 hours a day. This photograph was taken in the lounge at the Whippany headquarters. (Courtesy The Seeing Eye and Iris Veit.)

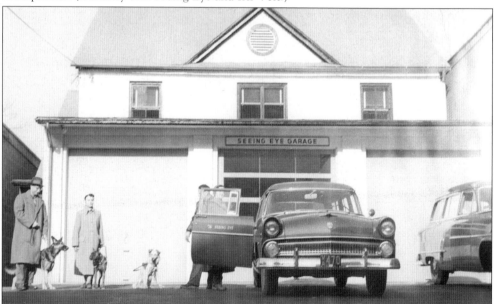

Although a student's first walk with the new dog is not easy, there is often a sense of invigoration. "Stepping out with the breathtaking new freedom of a tugging harness handle, students feel their backs and shoulders straighten, their lungs fill, their hearts beat," a graduate who experienced it explained. These students are about to leave the Whippany headquarters to train in Morristown. (Courtesy The Seeing Eye and Iris Veit.)

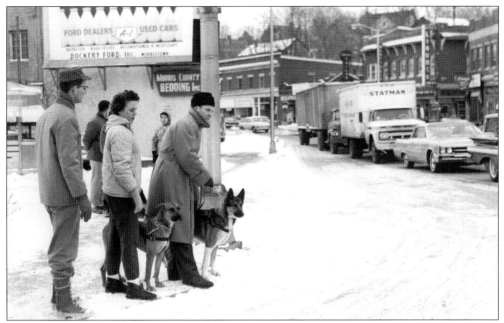

Training conditions can be invigorating as well. Although summer in Morristown is not as long and hot as it is in Nashville, winter can look like this. Students are put to the test in all kinds of situations, just as they might encounter in their hometowns. With the snow and the Morristown traffic, these students are getting their money's worth. (Courtesy The Seeing Eye and Dahlmeyer Studio.)

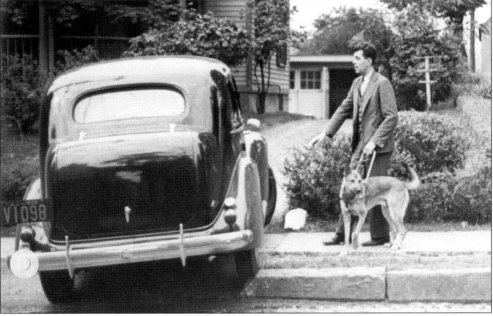

This is an example of intelligent disobedience in action. The master commanded the shepherd to go forward, not realizing that a car was about to turn in front of them. The dog correctly chose to disobey, stopping until the path cleared. Traffic-wise dogs learn to judge distances accurately so as not to endanger their masters.

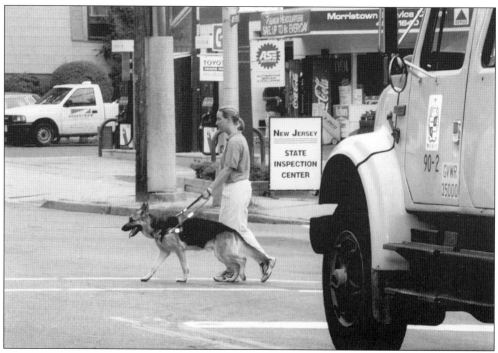

Dogs possess a unique desire to please humans. Other animals must be enticed by food or some other motivation to perform a task, while canines will often do it on the request of their master. Although dogs are considered intelligent, Jack Humphrey believed that their desire to please is what makes dogs most teachable.

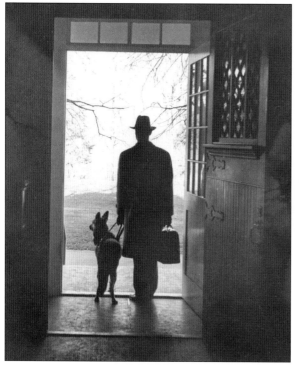

After witnessing a demonstration of Seeing Eye dogs in 1930, Helen Keller wrote to Dorothy Eustis, "Nothing hinders the spirit of usefulness more than inability to get about freely. . . . Lack of sight is not the terrible thing, but the thousand restraints it imposes. Through the work of The Seeing Eye, the burden of these restraints will be lightened, and the blind will, in some measure at least, be independent." (Courtesy The Seeing Eye and Nelson Groffman.)

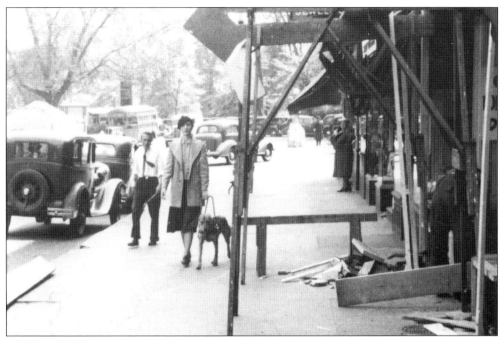

Students and their dogs first learn to work together in downtown Morristown, where the dogs have previously learned the routes. Afterward, training is tailored to the student's specific needs. An instructor will take an urban resident to New York City to learn to use the subway. A person who lives in the country is taught to walk along roads without sidewalks and curbs.

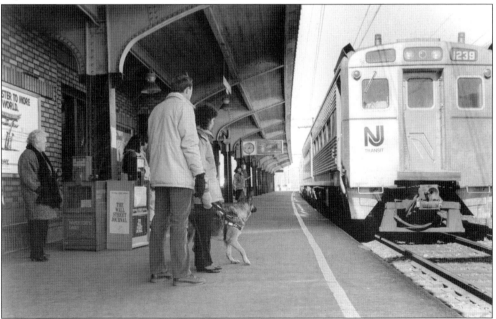

Subways and train stations have proven to be dangerous, especially when they are crowded. New Jersey Transit, with stations in Morristown and neighboring towns along the line, provides the opportunity for learning how to travel safely on trains. Many people who are blind live in cities to take advantage of public transportation and job opportunities.

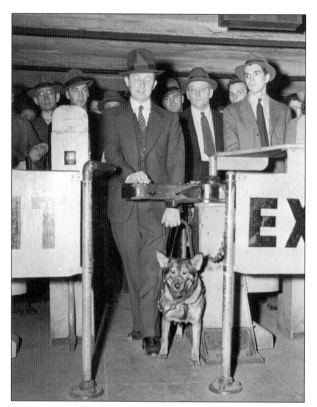

This graduate from many years ago is an example of a commuter on his way to work. He and his dog guide confidently walk through a turnstile in a crowded station. Most Seeing Eye graduates have a strong desire to stay active and move freely.

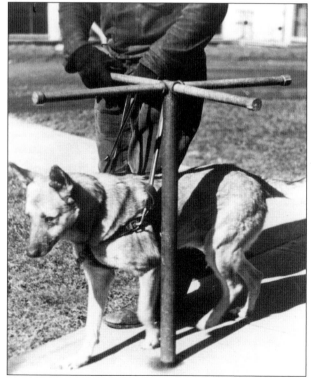

Turnstiles and revolving doors can be difficult for a person who cannot see. In many revolving doors, there is not much room for both person and dog, and more than one dog has caught its tail while trying to make it through. It takes some practice to master the skill. This photograph shows early turnstile training.

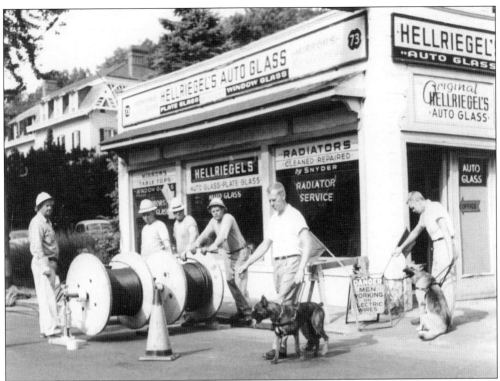

As life becomes more complicated, busier, and noisier, The Seeing Eye has had to adjust the students' and dogs' awareness of potential problems. Increased noise levels and quieter automobiles make it harder for people who are blind to hear and judge traffic. Newer automated traffic signals, such as green arrows for turns, complicate street crossings. These are several of the reasons that caused the school to increase the dog training period from three to four months.

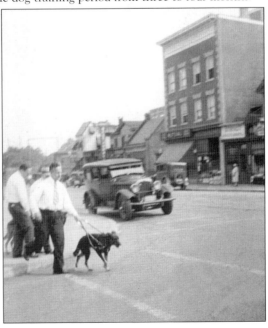

Since its founding in 1929, The Seeing Eye has stressed the point that sometimes well-meaning gestures by strangers can create dangerous situations for a blind person with a dog guide. Grabbing a person's arm, taking hold of the dog's harness, or shouting a warning can have the same effect as grabbing the steering wheel away from the driver of a moving car.

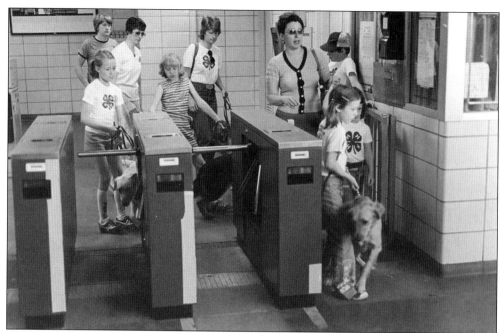

The Seeing Eye welcomes volunteering in many capacities. At any given time, 600 to 700 volunteers in New Jersey, Pennsylvania, and Delaware are raising Seeing Eye puppies. The program dates back to Switzerland in the late 1920s, when farmers were called on to help socialize Fortunate Fields' puppies. Jack Humphrey resurrected puppy raising in 1942 when he convinced the 4-H Club of Morris County to make puppy raising for The Seeing Eye one of its programs.

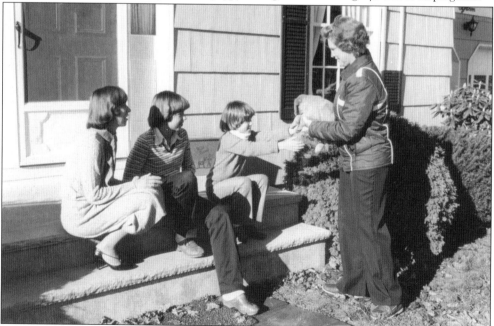

Puppies begin living with their puppy-raiser families when they are about eight weeks old and return to The Seeing Eye at about 18 months. They are then given aptitude tests; those that pass begin formal training.

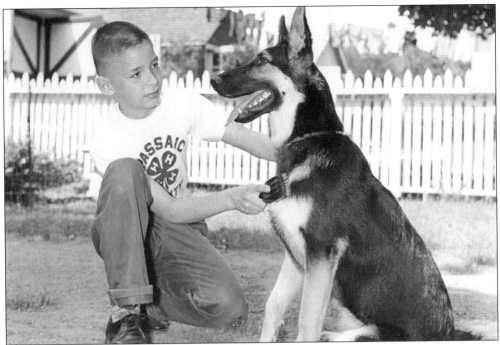

One person in the family takes primary responsibility for the puppy's daily care and routine, either a youngster between nine and 19, or an adult who is home during the day. Many retirees participate. The puppy is raised as a family member, taught basic obedience, and exposed to the kinds of situations it will encounter as a working dog. Love, stimulation, and socialization are key ingredients to good puppy raising.

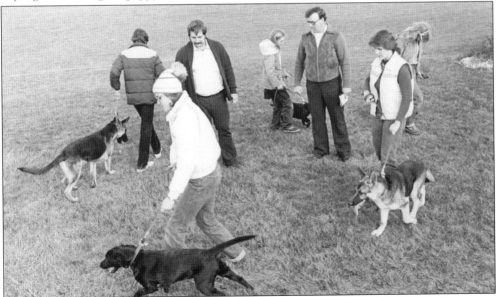

Although it is not necessary to belong to the 4-H to become a puppy raiser, volunteers agree to follow The Seeing Eye's puppy-raising curriculum and to attend regular club meetings with their puppies, as seen here. The Seeing Eye pays the veterinary bills and provides a stipend to defray puppy-related expenses.

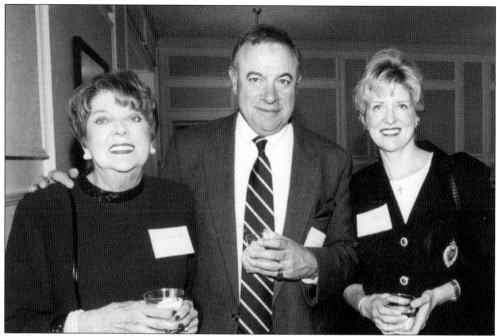

Volunteers support The Seeing Eye every day in many different ways. Dorothy Calderwood (left) is an example. Without her, this book would never have been possible. She spent years cataloguing the extensive Seeing Eye photograph and document archive. The Volunteer of the Year in 1999 is shown with Larry and Faith Amoroso, her son-in-law and daughter.

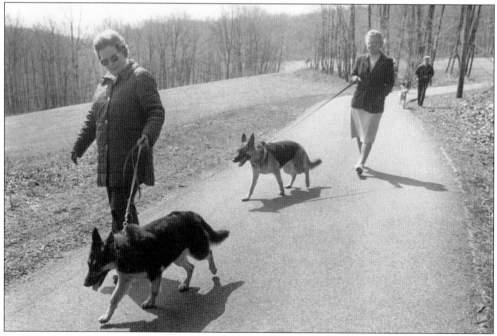

Georgie Little (left) became a volunteer dog walker in 1978 and is still going strong. Every Monday, she closes her yarn shop in Mendham to help exercise the dogs-in-training. She also bathes dogs just before they are matched with their new masters.

74

German shepherd Kristie—shown with her master, Blanche Carnes—is an example of what a Seeing Eye dog can do in a potentially life-threatening situation. There was a gas leak in the Carnes home one night; Kristie alerted the family, and they all escaped unharmed. For her heroism, Kristie received a medal of honor from William Rockefeller, president of the American Society for the Prevention of Cruelty to Animals. (Courtesy The Seeing Eye and Al Levine.)

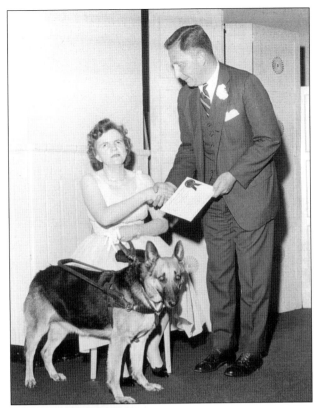

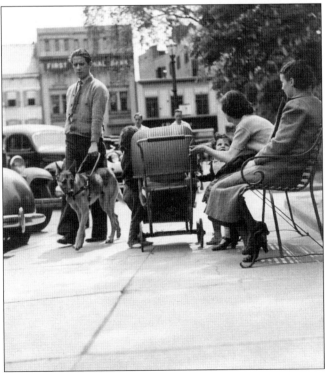

Tests from the 1950s showed that puppies whose socialization with humans was maintained from the first few weeks of life through their training period had a much greater chance of becoming successful guides, like the shepherd shown in this photograph. A mother's love and discipline during the first seven weeks of a puppy's life are also critical to successful development.

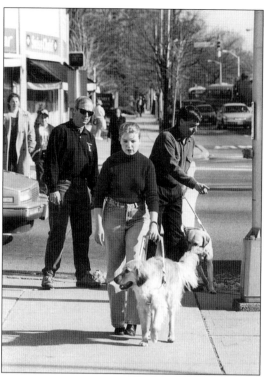

In the 1990s, The Seeing Eye reduced its student-to-instructor ratio from six to four students per instructor in order to provide a more individualized approach to learning. To accomplish this, The Seeing Eye steadily expanded its faculty, dog population, and infrastructure. An instructor (left) is shown with two students during their final week of class.

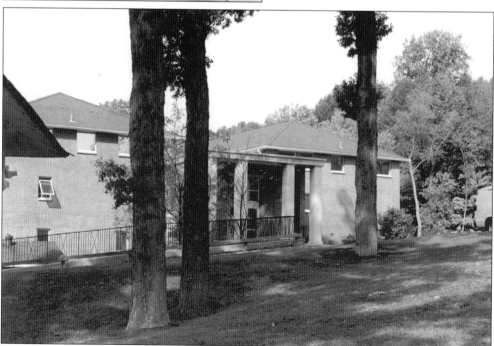

A major challenge faced by the philanthropy is the ability to accommodate the growing number of qualified students. An expansion program has been under way for more than a decade. One example of the planned growth and development is the Walker Dillard Kirby Canine Center, which opened on the Washington Valley campus in 1993. It houses 120 dogs-in-training.

Four

BUDDIES WITHOUT
BOUNDARIES

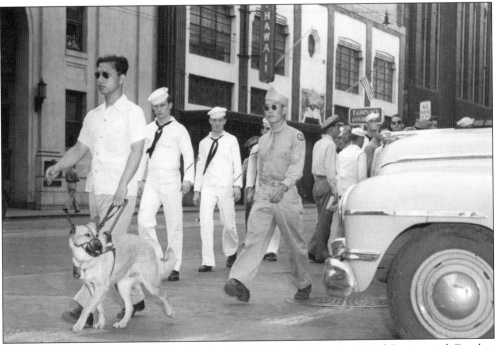

Yoshina Omiya was a private first class in the U.S. Army's famous 442nd Regimental Combat Team, composed of Americans of Japanese ancestry, when he was blinded during an assault on German-held Hill 600 in Italy in 1943. Thirteen months later, he was training at The Seeing Eye in Whippany with his German shepherd, Audrey. The buddies are shown here in Omiya's hometown of Honolulu. (Courtesy The Seeing Eye and the Signal Corps.)

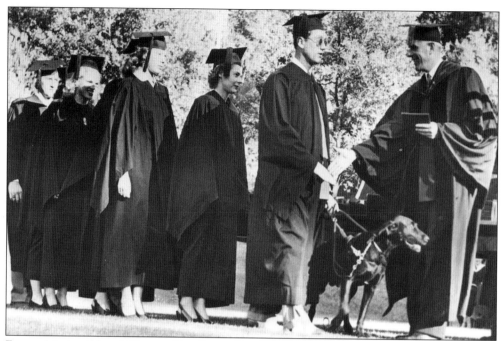

Former Marine Edward Glass and his Seeing Eye dog, Ruff, accept the student's bachelor of arts diploma during graduation ceremonies at Stanford University in the late 1940s. When university official Donald Tresidder (right) took a moment to pay tribute to Glass and Ruff, some 7,000 fellow graduates stood and applauded. (Courtesy The Seeing Eye and Acme Photo.)

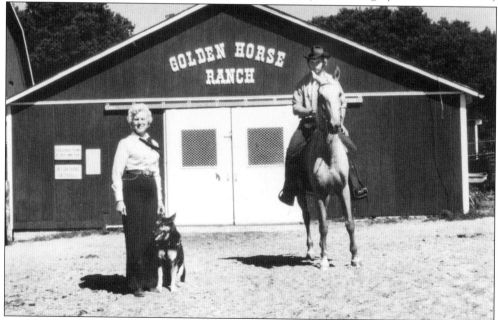

It often takes six months to a year for a Seeing Eye graduate and dog to become an accomplished team. If a problem develops, The Seeing Eye provides postgraduation assistance, including a visit to the home if the situation warrants. Graduate Ruth Coleman appears to be doing just fine back home on her ranch.

"Dogs offer students a kind of freedom they have rarely received from human guides," wrote graduate Peter Brock Putnam in his book about The Seeing Eye called *Love in the Lead*. Putnam, a graduate of The Seeing Eye and member of its board, also had a doctor of philosophy degree in history. He taught at Princeton University, authored several books, and served as national chairman of Recording for the Blind and Dyslexic. Putnam is shown here out for a walk with his ninth Seeing Eye dog, Pasha.

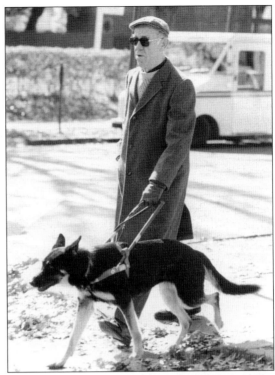

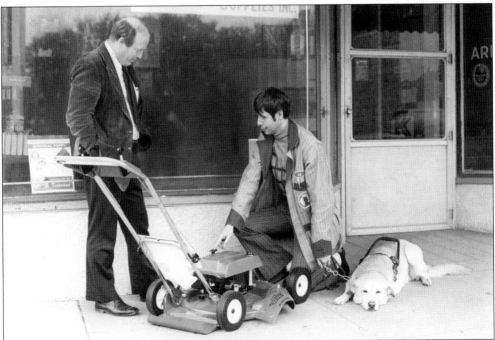

Graduates possess many types of skills and come from all walks of life. The average working life of a Seeing Eye dog is from eight to 10 years. After retirement, the dogs stay with their master, are adopted by friends or relatives, or are found a loving home by The Seeing Eye. (Courtesy The Seeing Eye and Jeff Notto.)

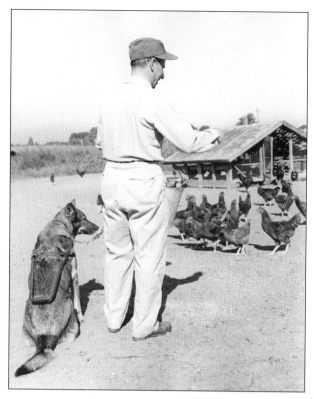

This man always worked close to the land. After losing his sight, he was not deterred. He graduated from The Seeing Eye and became a successful chicken farmer. Companion dogs allow many graduates the chance to lessen their dependency on family and friends. (Courtesy The Seeing Eye and Iris Veit.)

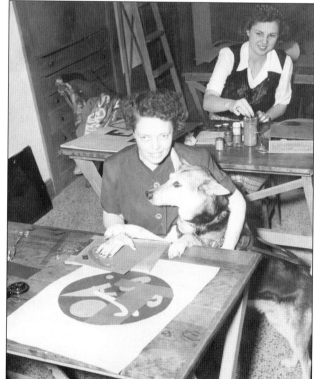

Genevieve Powell of Texas and guide Blackie are busy in the design laboratory at the Texas State College for Women in Denton. She used her design skills to work as an occupational therapist, helping others "worse off than myself."

John Stowall of West Point, Mississippi, takes a break from his job as a disc jockey at WROB. Dogs are unique in their emotional attachment to human beings. Even highly intelligent apes lack this type of psychological bond.

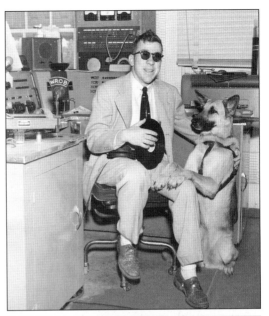

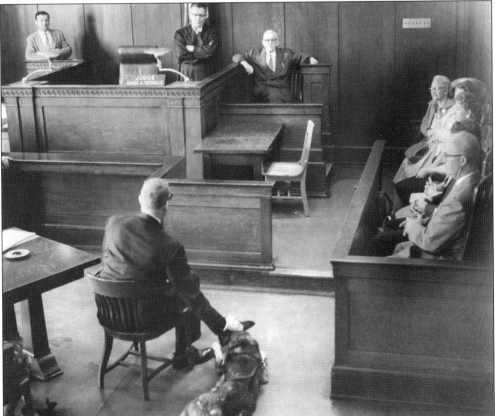

This graduate became an attorney. His partner sits in the courtroom next to him as he pleads his case before the judge and jury. Blindness imprisons some people. For many, Seeing Eye dogs offer freedom.

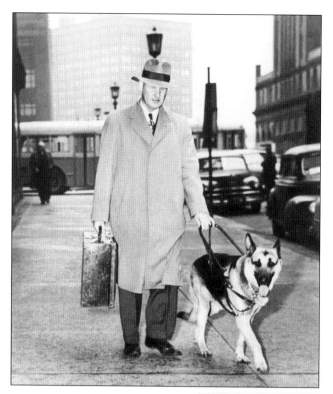

Anyone who has pounded the pavement on sales calls knows what a tough job that can be. This salesman and his guide are heading for their next appointment. Seeing Eye graduates can be found working alongside sighted persons in more than 100 occupations.

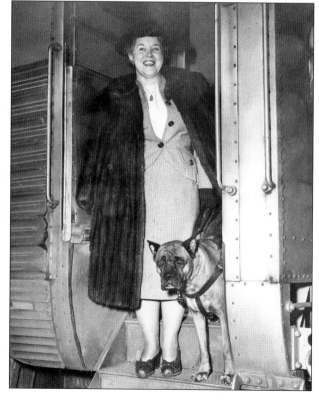

Norine McNichols of Chicago was a sales instructor. She and her boxer are on their way to teach retail employees effective selling techniques in 1948. Today, there are about 1,800 active Seeing Eye graduates. (Courtesy The Seeing Eye and the Los Angeles Times.)

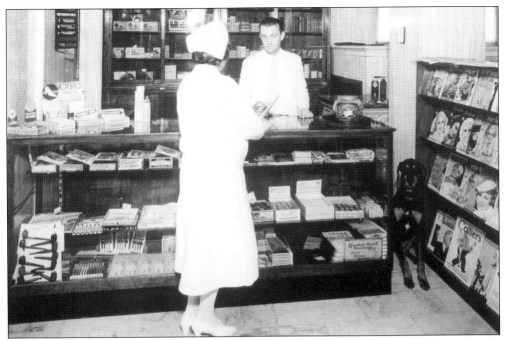

The dog guide at right was the first Seeing Eye Doberman pinscher. He went to work with master Ray Ulmer at his news and tobacco stand in Pennsylvania. The ability to be independent is what draws students to The Seeing Eye.

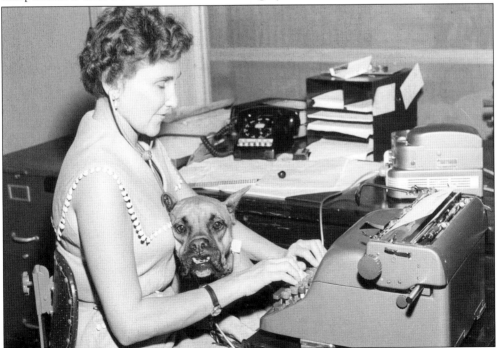

Most Seeing Eye graduates are gainfully employed or productive in other ways. This woman was a secretary whose boxer appeared to enjoy the job as much as the master. (Courtesy The Seeing Eye and Associated Photographers.)

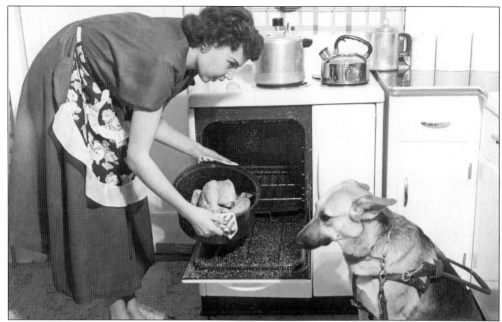

Some graduates are homemakers. It looks as though this shepherd had a moderate interest in the dinner menu that night. Seeing Eye dogs are technically not pets. They are working dogs that are carefully trained to guide people during their daily activities. (Courtesy The Seeing Eye and Rue Studio.)

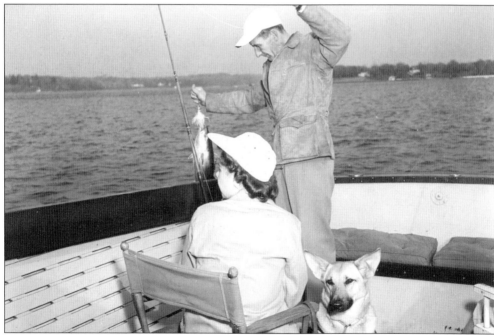

In addition to work, there is also time for recreation. This graduate and his wife try their luck at fishing while the guide takes in the salt air. Helping people who are blind and visually impaired remain active has always been a goal of The Seeing Eye. (Courtesy The Seeing Eye and Rue Studio.)

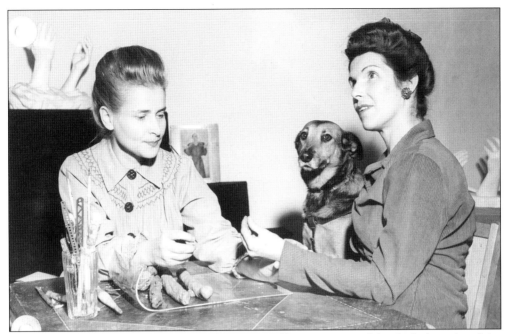

Graduate Dorothy Schrier (right) is in the process of being recognized for the helping hand she provided to the war effort during World War II. A model of her hands is being sculpted by Ray Shaw for a special exhibit at Madison Square Garden that paid tribute to America's women war workers. Her dog, Lorn, keeps an eye on the session. Schrier worked in a New Jersey defense plant. (Courtesy The Seeing Eye and Hope Associates.)

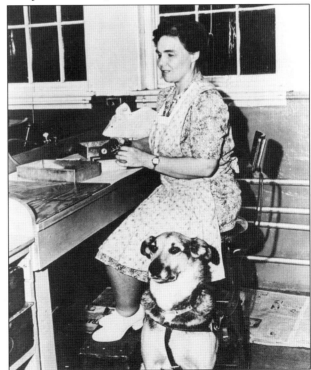

This graduate also contributed to the war effort. She worked as an inspector in a factory that produced firing pins for time fuses. Many Seeing Eye graduates were employed in defense-related industries during World War II.

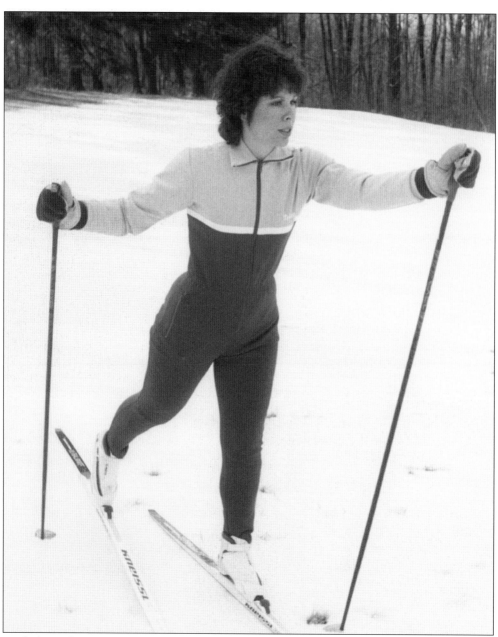

Michele Drolet measures up to the standards that Seeing Eye pioneers envisioned when they began. As a member of the U.S. Disabled Cross Country Ski Team, she brought home the bronze medal in the five-kilometer freestyle event at the Paralympic Winter Games in Lillehammer, Norway, in 1994. Drolet became the first American female athlete, disabled or able-bodied, to win a medal in Olympic cross-country skiing. Paralympic games are held on the same courses as the Olympic games after the Olympics conclude. Legally blind since birth, Drolet started downhill skiing at age four and later switched to cross-country. She trained with her first Seeing Eye dog in 1974, when she decided it would be a good idea to study in Paris. Now with a master's degree, Drolet is the student relations manager at The Seeing Eye, working with students and graduates on issues and concerns they face.

A.J. Bell of Austin, Texas, collects the check at his lunch counter in 1965. His dog, Candy, keeps an eye on the transaction. "We here are not The Seeing Eye," Willi Ebeling once said. "The Seeing Eye is not the staff or this building. The Seeing Eye is the graduates and their dogs out in the field."

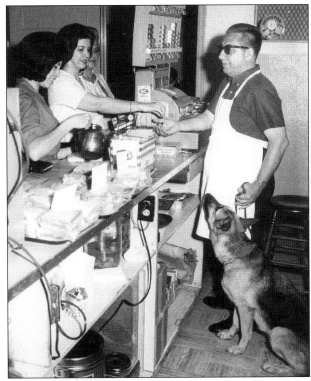

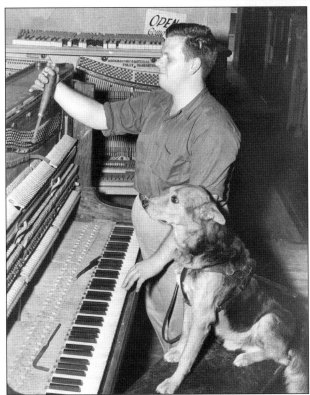

Although this team is gainfully employed and doing just fine, some graduates experience difficulties when they first leave The Seeing Eye. It can take time for a graduate to commit unwavering trust to a dog. Occasionally, dogs do not follow their masters' commands as they did during training. Some dogs become spoiled when they get home, which can hinder performance. On rare occasions, graduates discover that a dog guide is not for them.

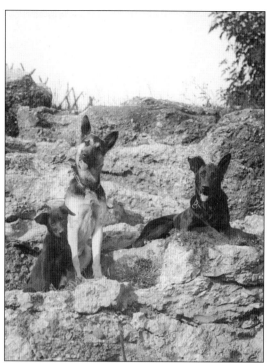

Although somewhat perplexing, jealousy has created problems for several graduates. From as long ago as the 1930s, there have been incidents when dogs have been returned because a spouse of a recent graduate would become jealous of the new dog or the loved one's newfound freedom. (Courtesy The Seeing Eye and A. Dauer.)

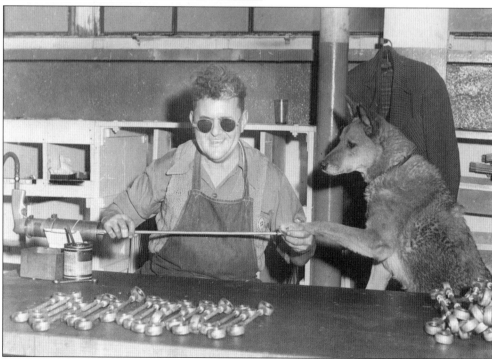

In addition to caring for a dog's physical needs, a master must also provide emotional support—demonstrating concern, affection, as well as trust in his companion. This makes for a true partnership. Graduate Bill Hassett and his dog, Pal, appear to have mastered the partnership concept.

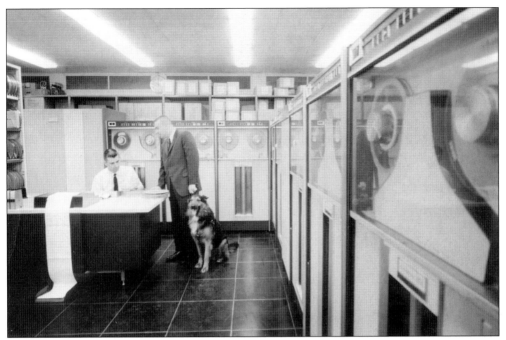

Computers have come a long way in recent decades, but Seeing Eye programs have remained essentially the same since 1929. The principle of independence and dignity for those who are blind and visually impaired is as important today in Morristown as it was in Vevey.

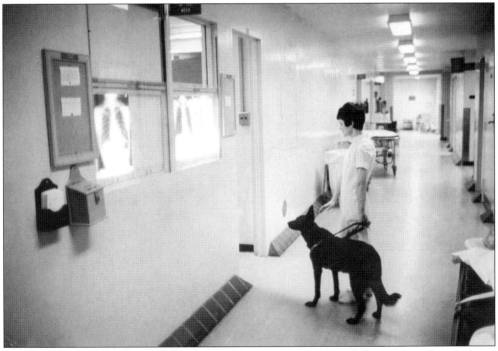

Many graduates have worked in the healthcare industries, including hospital technician Marilyn Rodda (shown here). Some Seeing Eye graduates have reported that it was their dogs that provided the positive reinforcement they needed to return to gainful employment.

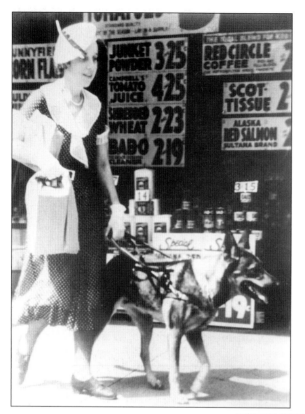

Although stopping at the grocery store to pick up dinner is a routine event for sighted people, it is not something that a person who is blind gets a chance to do every day—unless, of course, a person has a Seeing Eye dog. With her right arm filled with groceries and the left hand holding the harness, this graduate heads for home.

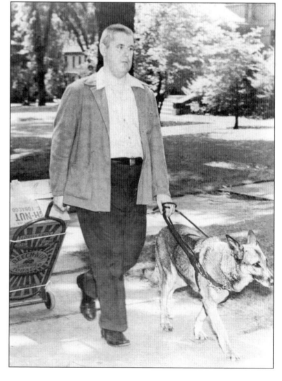

When he needed supplies for the canteen he operated at a company in Syracuse, New York, Bob Dinet harnessed his dog, Chen, grabbed a hand truck, and headed to the wholesaler to pick them up. It was a long haul they had to make several times a week, but Dinet took it in stride.

George Risko was the first blind probation officer in the United States, according to the Juvenile Court of Allegheny County (Pennsylvania). He and his dog, Gretchen, worked there with youngsters who had gotten into trouble. "Children respond well to Gretchen," Risko explained. "She helps improve the relationship between me and the child." Risko, who lost his sight as a young child, studied at Pennsylvania State University and the University of Pittsburgh, earning a bachelor's and a master's degree. (Courtesy The Seeing Eye and Edwin Morgan, Sun-Telegraph.)

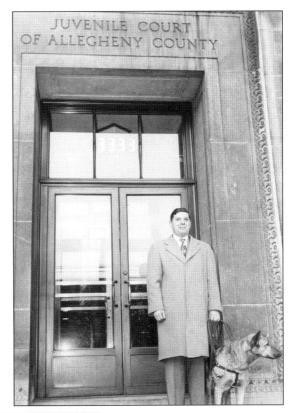

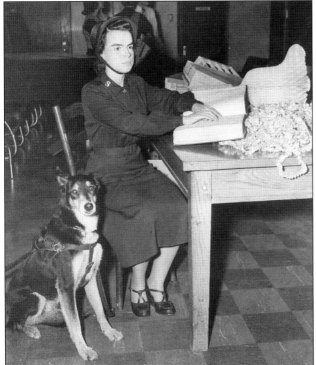

Another humanitarian who was supported by a dog guide was Norma Claypoole, shown reading a Braille Bible with Dutchess by her side. Claypoole was a member of the Salvation Army. In fact, she wrote Christmas carols in Braille that were performed by the group during the holiday season.

91

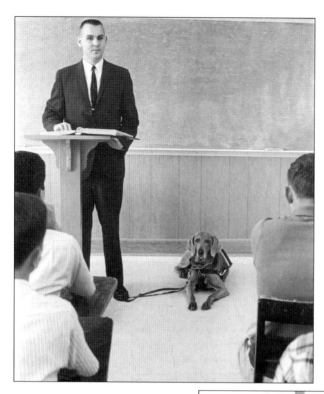

Many Seeing Eye graduates are highly educated. Dr. Otis Stephens was a professor of political science at Georgia Southern College in Statesboro. He is shown lecturing as Lady keeps tabs on the collegians.

A sniper's bullet on Okinawa blinded Marine Edward Hoyczyk during World War II, but it did not stop him. The Buffalonian went on to earn a bachelor of arts degree with the help of his Seeing Eye dog, Jay. Hoyczyk advanced his education at the Harvard Graduate School of Business. The Seeing Eye had provided dogs for 163 veterans by 1950, and the organization continues to serve them with dogs to this day.

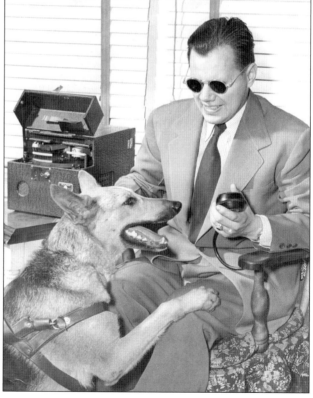

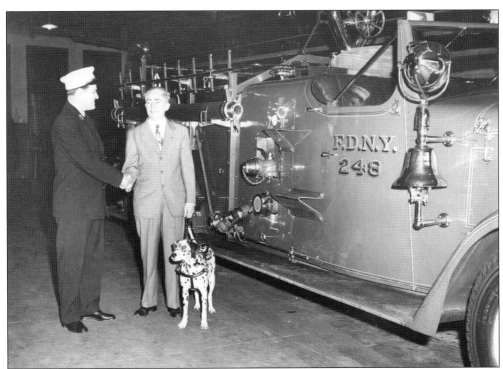

Dog guide Cinder was named the official mascot for Engine Company No. 248 of the New York Fire Department c. 1950. She is shown at the station house with her master, William White of Brooklyn. Cinder was also the mascot for the American Legion Post No. 930 of the New York Fire Department. (Courtesy The Seeing Eye and the New York Fire Department; Heavey photographer.)

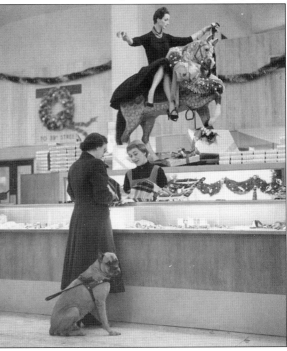

Although her boxer looks like he would rather be home watching football, Elsie Teplensky enjoys an afternoon of Christmas shopping in 1955. "It is the most wonderful sensation to go quickly where I want to go, depending on no one, and knowing all the time that I shall get there safely," Morris Frank explained soon after coming home with Buddy.

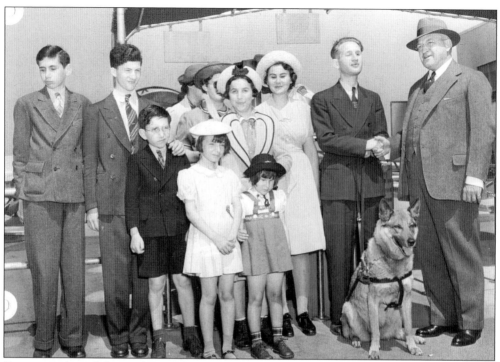

Despite a rule prohibiting dogs, the 1940 World's Fair in New York allowed 10-year-old Seeing Eye dog Zenta to visit the fairgrounds with her master, Carl Weiss. Weiss is shown shaking hands with Harvey Gibson, chairman of the board of the fair. The children who joined in on the fun were from the Home of the New York Guild for the Jewish Blind.

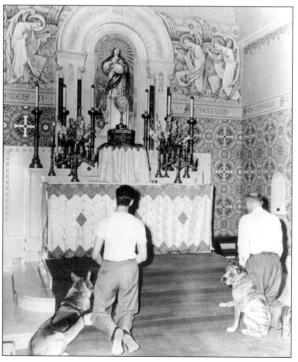

Seeing Eye dogs accompany their masters to houses of worship throughout the United States and Canada. A number of graduates are members of the clergy. Rev. R.A. Blair wrote more than 70 years ago that his Seeing Eye dog, Dot, "took me to church, Sabbath morning, and lay at my feet in the pulpit while I preached from the text."

The horizon is virtually endless for some graduates. In the 1930s, The Seeing Eye sent a questionnaire to its graduates asking, among other things, for comments on their dogs' services. One person responded by saying that the dog guide "rebuilds in the individual the joy of living."

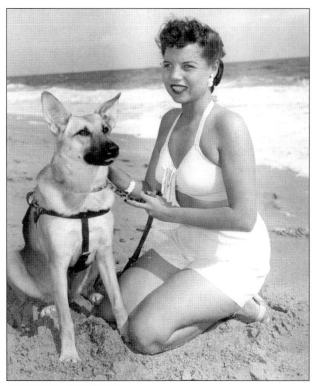

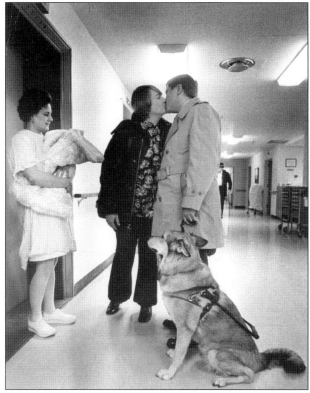

Seeing Eye dogs sometimes get the chance to experience very special moments. A newborn baby is shown heading home to join a growing family. Meanwhile, the mission of educating dogs as reasoning, safe, and efficient guides to the blind and visually impaired continues.

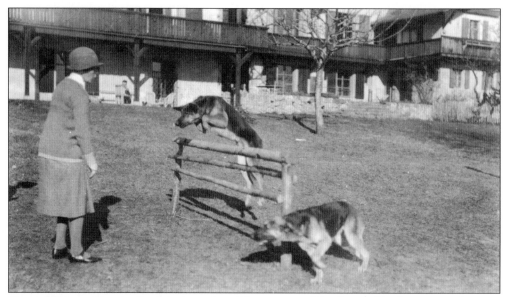

Since its conception in Europe more than 70 years ago, The Seeing Eye has matured into a respected philanthropy. Dorothy Harrison Eustis (shown at Fortunate Fields in the 1920s) would have been pleased with the results of her creation. She said during a radio interview in 1933, "If it lay within your power to give eyes to the blind—eyes which would enable thousands of them to go through traffic, to move with freedom from place to place, to go from one city to another or anywhere, in fact, that they cared to go—if this lay within your power, would you do it? We, of The Seeing Eye, have been fortunate enough to have had an opportunity of this kind, and as far as we have been able, we have grasped it." (Below courtesy The Seeing Eye and George Diehl.)

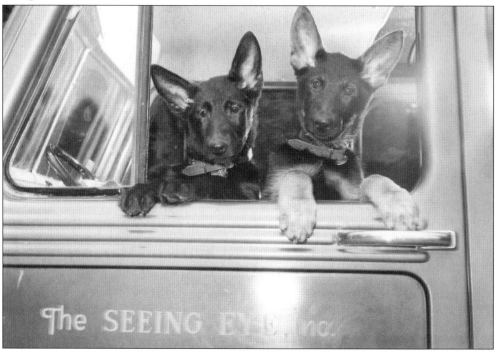